Michael Morgan

The Secret Life of Crohn's
Growing up with a Hidden Disease

Copyright © 2025 Michael Morgan
All rights reserved.

No part of this book may be reproduced or transmitted by any means or in any form,
except as permitted by UK copyright law or the author.
This book does not constitute medical, legal or other actionable advice.

Illustrated by mrgrubbson

ISBN: 978-1-3999-9762-1

For the secret sufferers

Table of Contents

The C-Word	*1*
Tummy Trouble	*3*
OUT OF ORDER	*8*
Teenager Crohnicles	*17*
The Crohn Ranger	*29*
FOOD FIGHT!!	*37*
Gut Outta Here	*43*
Ileostomy, Myself and I	*51*
A New Life?	*56*
A New Life!	*67*
All Crohn Up	*77*
Mental Flares	*93*
No More Secrets	*97*

Appendix

Parental Guidance	*105*
Dating Crohn's	*119*

- The C-Word -

Diagnosed aged ten, my story traverses the difficulties that this easily misunderstood illness brings to children, teenagers and young adults - from school, diet and treatment, to relationships, sex and living with an ostomy bag.

In the last 22 years this disease has affected my life in many ways, good and bad. The hardships can feel incredibly unfair and distressing, but I want to assure you it is possible to get through them and come out stronger, with a new perspective on life. Looking back now many memories are shocking, but eventually you accept and even see the funny side of the embarrassing situations that inevitably come with Crohn's Disease.

I don't hold back in this record of my experiences, so be prepared for some accounts of a more graphic nature. Please don't feel bad at laughing at some of the crappy situations this illness has put me in, I certainly do.

Crohn's Disease and Ulcerative Colitis are the most notorious Inflammatory Bowel Diseases (IBD) - not to be confused with Irritable Bowel Syndrome (IBS). Crohn's and Colitis are both long-term chronic conditions affecting the digestive system with inflammation - Colitis is confined to the large intestine, but Crohn's can be active anywhere from top to bottom, mouth to anus.

There is a wide spectrum of severity within these diseases, with some cases being easily managed, but in others the conditions can be very tenacious, with years of constant flare-ups and only short periods of real control or remission. Unfortunately, I am one of the latter cases. For eight years my family and I struggled through my adolescence, exhausting all treatments, from steroids, immunosuppressants and biological injections, to suppositories, enemas and a strict liquid diet, until the only option left was surgery.

Although an unhealthy childhood is not the cheeriest of topics to read about, I hope that the later chapters can offer reassurance, to people and families who are troubled by these diseases, that a more than completely normal life is possible.

My intention is for this book to increase the understanding of the human side of IBD, giving a frank insight into the more unseen aspects of facing up to the symptoms and trials of these aggressive illnesses.

The appendix chapters step away from my vantage point and offer an alternative perspective on the disease; shining a light on what it is like to have an unwell child, and exposing some of the obstacles of being in a relationship with a Crohn's sufferer.

- Tummy Trouble -

I remember going to the toilet more often and for much longer. There were these new pains in my belly, that would briefly go away when on the toilet, but always came back. I didn't understand it, this wasn't like the other times I had been poorly. Had I done something bad? Did I not eat enough vegetables?

This continued for weeks, as a ten-year-old I had no concept that this was an indicator of real health problems. Just like a cough or a cold, surely this would stop soon. There was no need for anyone to know - especially as I had been hiding it for a while now. The clearest memory I have from this inception period is the first time I saw the blood, such a bright vivid colour on the toilet tissue. This was shocking, but more than anything confusing. The strangeness of the red water intensified the secret. Concealing whatever was happening felt normal, the bloody toilet bowl became routine. I turned it into a game, the 'hiding game'. Sneaking to the bathroom and thinking of excuses for why I was in there for so long. 'I'm just playing my Gameboy', or 'I'm just getting a tissue' or just plainly denying that I was in there at all. I had thought that going to the toilet multiple times an hour - until my legs went numb - was normal, and that everyone else was just very good at the game.

My increasing paleness, and the hours spent in the bathroom were not unnoticed by my mum, but the explicit warnings were hidden behind a locked toilet door. Fortunately, my sharp weight loss was a tell-tale sign and 'Is everything ok?' quickly became 'What is going on?! You have to tell me what is happening!'

'Nothing!' would be the response as my natural stubbornness would not budge. The despair in my parents' questions only exposed the upsetting truth that I would have to face up to what the blood and pain were telling me, making me sink further into my cover up and desperate denial.

Despite my best efforts, 'enough was enough' and I was dragged to see the local doctor. We were told there was nothing major to worry about, it was simply gastroenteritis, which should clear up in a week or so - my paleness was just my skin tone.

No food was staying inside me, what I had previously thought of as stealthy endeavours - slipping unnoticed to the toilet during mealtimes - were now all too apparent to my family. After a few more days at home, it was more than clear to my mum that this was not normal for a ten-year-old boy, something had to be done. I was marched back, kicking and screaming, to the doctor's office. My parents' hysteria was met with appeasing statements like 'these things can take a while' and 'just wait and see'. Regardless, my insistent mum demanded further action and a stool sample was requested.

There was no way to hide it now. My mum's shock at the amount of blood was matched by the hospital staff upon handing the sample in. I was admitted that day.

This was the first time I had stayed in hospital; I was lucky to be given my own room with a personal bathroom attached. I didn't really understand what was going on, it felt like I was in trouble, but people were being so nice to me. Things moved very fast, there were all kinds of samples taken and many questions - not just from the doctors. I went into my shell when a nurse or doctor came into the room, responding to their questions via my parents or mumbling the answers - I wanted to go home. It was no doubt an extremely worrisome period for my family, but there was relief in that now there would be some answers.

It is strange the things that you remember most clearly; I somewhat recall that my throat and bum were sore after my first scopes (colonoscopy and endoscopy*), but I can vividly recall my first encounter with pre-procedure preparations. An enema - at that age - is of course daunting and unnerving, but the bowel-prep was the real nemesis. You drink at least a litre of the stuff (mine was called Picolax) over several hours to clear out your system - not that mine needed a helping hand - to ensure the cameras have a clear view. It seems somewhat trivial now, but at the time that murky pink jug was a mountain to climb. It goes without saying that this stuff is tough to stomach, but it is the unpalatable, chemical smell that has stuck with me.

My teacher came to visit me that day - bringing get-well-soon cards from my school friends. She shrewdly invented a way of getting me to drink it. We played a game, and when I won a hand of cards, I would have to take a sip - she knew I could not ignore my competitive nature and that I couldn't argue with her like I could with my parents.

Eventually enough was forced down and it worked its magic before the cameras went in the following morning. You do get as much ice cream and jelly as you want when you wake up from the anaesthetic, which is always nice. Picolax was later added to my medicine allergy list - on the third or fourth colonoscopy - following a full night of stomach pains and dry retching every 15 minutes. I *really* hate that stuff.

The scope results were interpreted as Ulcerative Colitis (later the diagnosis was changed to Crohn's Disease). At this time (2002) Inflammatory Bowel Disease was rare in younger children; because of this and the severity of the findings I was referred to a specialist paediatric gastroenterology team in a central London hospital.

I had no concept of what Ulcerative Colitis was or what that meant for me, no way to process or understand it - other than my experience of the symptoms and the word 'ulcer'... which didn't sound very nice. The diagnosis was really for my parents, it brought reprieve that it wasn't something more serious, but also a truth and realisation that this wasn't going to be over in a few weeks.

Colonoscopy – following heavy duty laxatives and a rinsing enema, a small camera is passed up the bottom to examine the rectum and the whole large bowel. As well as the visuals – for example of inflammation and ulcerations – biopsies can be taken to aid diagnosis. Adults are usually partially sedated or kept awake for the procedure, but children are typically fully anesthetised.

Endoscopy – similar to a colonoscopy, but instead the camera goes down the throat to inspect the upper part of the digestive tract.

- OUT OF ORDER -

Things were now out in the open with a clearer idea of what was going on, but it was still a very bewildering time. My life had changed. In a month or two my fairly normal childhood was over. I hadn't been to school in weeks; my time was now split between being at home and visiting the hospital. I wasn't housebound as such, but leaving the house was extremely stressful.

The toilet seat became my safe place, it was a place that pain was relieved and somewhere my brain could rest from the constant bathroom related worries. 'Where is the nearest toilet?', 'What would I do if I needed to go right now?' and 'Is there enough toilet roll in there?'

As my disease was mostly active on the lower end of the digestive tract, this meant that I had almost no warning time, I could go from feeling perfectly content, to having 10-20 seconds before a messy accident was going to happen. There was no 'holding it in', the pain was too much.

The one expedition I could not argue against was the dreaded hospital appointments. Not dreaded because I was afraid, or didn't particularly like answering doctors' questions, or listening to them and my parents talk about me, but because of the journey itself. My debilitating need to be within 10 seconds of a toilet, made this quite simple trip 60 minutes of pure anxiety and terror. A tube train full of strangers is unquestionably near the top of 'worst places to desperately need the loo'. Another that comes to mind is on an airplane when the seat belt sign is on. Anyway, I'm your man if you need someone to tell you every station on the

Piccadilly line which has a public toilet in or around it. Now there's an idea for an app!

The major problem was that I couldn't eat, or keep anything down. My body rejected food, one way or the other. An incessant cycle ensued - struggling to eat, followed by either winning or losing a race to the toilet, and then not wanting to eat again afterwards. Vomiting added the occasional variation to the toilet trips, sometimes it was the rotting, gag inducing smell of my poo that would trigger it (we would joke there was something dying inside of me), but more commonly it was the pain that was just too much to bear. Usually throwing-up almost immediately brought an end to it, or at least to that round.

Abdominal pain is the most glaring physical symptom of Crohn's. The spells of pain were usually unpredictable, but whenever I ate, I knew it wouldn't be long before I would have to withdraw into myself to contain it. I would go quiet and people learnt not to engage with me.

It can be sudden, short and sharp - catching you off guard and stopping you in your tracks, it can be irritatingly dull and constant, or more often than not, the worst of both worlds - coming in consistent waves for an extended period, usually building up and up and up.

Imagine you have a bleeding graze on your arm, the area becomes swollen and more sensitive to touch. Now someone comes and presses sand paper on the cut and starts rubbing it. This is how I describe the worst pains. The sandpaper is faecal matter, scraping long sections of your wounded and already irritated insides. The intense burning and grinding lasting a minute or so, subsiding and then recommencing.

It was clear that school wasn't going to be an option for a while - I missed nearly all of Year 5 of primary school. My mum was forced to quit her job to look after me at home. Here began a treatment cycle that continued until I was 17 years-old, it went;

1. A new treatment or an increase in the dosage
2. Wait to see if it has an effect (if not back to step 1)
3. Remission or reasonable control for a month or two (if we were lucky)
4. The treatment's effectiveness would dwindle
5. Relapse and repeat

The dose and power of the drugs prescribed were incrementally increased in an attempt to reach a level of stability. There is a reluctance to jump straight in with the most powerful medicines – as if it is at all possible it makes sense to avoid these stronger drugs, which potentially bring more severe side-effects and additional future complications.

As well as this, it can take a while for a new drug (or a new dosage) to build-up to the desired levels in your system. This is then followed by a waiting game to see if there is any improvement… and then back to the hospital to reassess. Therefore, Stage 1 and 2 in the above cycle often took a very long time, many months before there was any real change.

This is the only appropriate approach, but the delay between the tweaks to the treatment plan and feeling the results was very frustrating and exhausting. Sometimes I knew a small dose increase wasn't going to help, but this was the procedure.

I do not know if this is still the medical thinking, but there was a belief that children would 'grow out of Crohn's', not as in cured, but that once the body settles down after puberty and growing, there was a mellowing of the disease - with the symptoms being more easily regulated. So the challenge we faced was seeing through the havoc of childhood and adolescence, and avoiding treatments that can have lasting ramifications – such as steroids and surgery.

The baseline treatment was a cocktail of anti-inflammatories and immunosuppressants - inflammation is an immune system's response, so weakening this in theory lowers inflammation. On top of this was drinking Modulen - a nutritional support drink. A diseased gut doesn't digest or absorb well - with the internal lining being inflamed, ulcerated and generally damaged. This drink became a part of my diet when things began to go downhill, but better nourishment provided little comfort when things fell off a cliff.

The safety net to catch these steep relapses, and the only medication that worked swiftly and magically for me was steroids (Prednisolone). Within a week or two of starting a course my appetite would improve and some colour would return to my face. The biggest miracle was that after a few weeks I would pass solid stools - the first plop was met with cheer and celebrated like Christmas. I would briefly become a normal, chubby little boy, a stark contrast to the default walking skeleton - so pale I was almost see-through.

The wonder drug, however, has side effects which children are particularly susceptible to. There are potentially serious longer-term consequences such as stunted growth. The drug messes with your body's natural hormone balances, and growth hormone treatment is a whole new battle we didn't want to bring into the arena. As I was already walking along the lower edge of the 'normal range' on the Age vs Height graph, there was a strong reluctance to be prescribed steroids for any significant period of time; because of this I could only have a few blissful weeks of feeling 'normal'.

In these periods of adequate health, I still was reluctant to attend school. One reason was because of another side effect of Prednisolone - 'Moon-face' or 'Pred-head'. The medication as well as rapid weight gain can cause children's faces to swell. Picture a hamster or a squirrel with both cheeks stuffed with food.

The physical change can be quite dramatic, but I am sure it wasn't just the self-consciousness that kept me at home (children - at that time anyway - were not too concerned with appearances). My confidence was gone, the stress and isolation had naturally made me depressed, being at home was safe, being at home was my main comfort.

The routine of 'relapse, remission, repeat' continued through the summer. I remember the family holiday was cancelled and one eventful play-date that in hindsight was a real foreshadowing event for the next decade of my life.

My little-school best friend was having friends over, and not having seen any in a while, I was persuaded to go. The fact I had been to his house before was key. I knew there was a working toilet there… these things had to be seen to be believed, 'of course there will be a toilet there!' doesn't cut it. Thankfully it was just me, him and two other classmates. At some point it was decided we all were going to the park to play football, us children, his older brother and the parents. Now, this was quite a sticky situation, what could I do? I had no plausible excuse that would allow me to keep my illness and symptoms relatively secret and persuade everyone that in fact playing football in the park was a terrible idea.

How could his parents really understand my situation? Even if they had suspected that it would be difficult for me or that I wouldn't want to go, they probably did not consider the fact that I would not want to express this out loud… so we set off on a leisurely 20-minute walk to a vast green open space that I had not been to before. The stuff of Crohn's nightmares.

Inevitably, I needed the toilet. I stopped playing and gingerly walked over to his mum who was watching from the side. I asked if there was a toilet here. There wasn't. I stayed beside her clenching like my life depended on it. This is the pinnacle of pain for Crohn's, using the sandpaper / open wound analogy, this is like a sanding machine has fallen onto the cut. Unexpectedly, I weathered the storm and the urge subsided. From experience I knew that I had been very lucky here, this was a real rarity. Yet, I was still not out of the woods,

I didn't have a reason to not be playing football. Any movement increases the risk of needing to go, but I surmised that I didn't need to go right now, and that we had been there a while so must be heading back soon. Very shortly after resuming, I felt a clunk inside. I knew straight away there was no holding this in. There were no trees close enough and nothing to hide behind. I expressed that I needed to go, and sprinted away from where we were playing. This was my first public calamity. My panicked attempts to get my bottoms down had just about worked, but I had forgotten about the front end.

The hilariously bad smell was a good distraction for the boys, as I squelched back and explained to the mum that I had urinated on myself. She took me back to the house where I showered and was given clean clothes. In the shower I remember fearing that this would haunt me.

Even though I bet this was a highly laughable episode for any child - seeing a friend squatting in an open field about 20 metres away - it was never mentioned again.

A less messy memory I have from that year was clearing the school playground. I can picture the dinner ladies' angry and confused faces as they herded the kids off the tarmac. Exclaiming 'Who has done that!?', 'Someone has let something off' … assuming a stink bomb must have been dropped. Amongst the giggles came 'Miss, I think it was Michael', 'Don't be silly!' was the sharp reply as surely it wasn't possible for a little boy to produce such a potent and wide-spreading smell.

When Year 6 (the final year of primary school) came around I attended school sporadically. I spend most of the year plumped up on Modulen and steroids - as this was still pre-teen years the dangers of taking these were not yet at their peak. The really difficult times were still to come, as the security steroids had granted me, would turn into a balancing act of short-term gain vs long-term consequences. A clue to the outcome of this contest is that I am 5ft 6…and a bit.

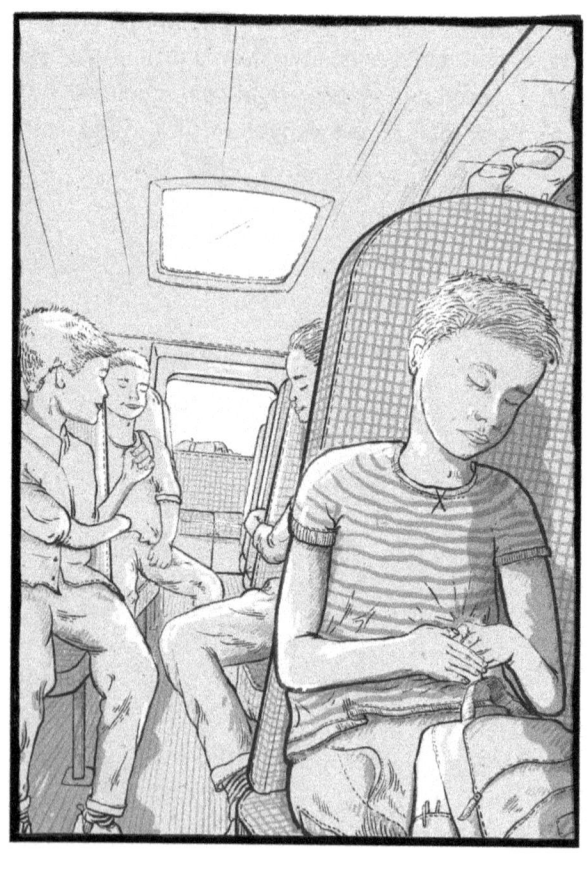

- Teenage Crohnicles -

It was time to start at a new school, being chained to the toilet was not really an option anymore, I had to try to get on with things. The internal debate that my mind wrestled with had now matured from worrying where the nearest toilet was / would be, to what steps can I take to reduce the risk of an accident on any public outing - as my now widening world had too many unforeseeable variables to adequately plan for.

The morning commute on the school bus was the embodiment of this. It was my behemoth. The first half of the day was always the more animated. I theorise that it is because overnight your system isn't stimulated giving it time to relax, clear out, and hopefully heal; and then when it is abruptly awoken by breakfast the hostility ensues - for me this was usually until about 2pm.

My primary school did not have a school bus, I was used to the stability, flexibility and reliability of being dropped off and picked up by a family member. This new challenge of a shaky, slow-moving vehicle full of older, louder, brazen children needed careful planning and preparation.

This would start the night before; not eating too late (to ensure my bowels had time to fully empty by the morning) and making sure there wasn't going to be any unexpected things to do that could disrupt my morning's strict schedule, such as an unpacked bag. I would get up extremely early and rush downstairs for breakfast, this was to give the food as long as possible to somewhat settle in my stomach. Then I would wake up my mum to give me my medicinal foam enema (until

I was old enough to do it myself), this was then followed by about 2 hours of concentrating on monitoring my tummy, and massaging it in an attempt to force through the digestion process. The last 40 minutes - up until the very last second - before I had to leave to walk (the motion of running would be too risky) to the bus stop was designated to sitting on the downstairs toilet (this gave me an extra 20 seconds as it was closer to the front door than the upstairs one). Here I pushed as hard as I possibly could, straining until I could see stars, in an attempt to get anything and everything out. I guess the thinking was - the less in there, the less that could go in my pants.

Even with my best laid plans, there were many days I knew getting off the toilet just wasn't an option, and numerous times I would be waiting at the bus stop and just have to walk home - much to the confusion of the other pupils, inevitably resulting in a full and thorough inquest the following day.

Once on the bus, things were generally ok - I wouldn't have got on if I wasn't 99.9% sure I would make it to school unsoiled. I even had a creative way of sitting; I would lean on one butt cheek and then subtly push the other into it with my hand and then roll back onto both, this meant my weight was self-clenching my cheeks - every little helps. This was how I started my school day for six years; but it was just the beginning of the daily campaign.

The next complication was the condition of the school's toilet blocks. It was a case of same shit, different much dirtier, likely blocked or vandalised, very much public toilet. Each day the terrain would change, which toilet seats were intact and useable, and which toilet blocks were not out-of-order. Once a somewhat applicable cubicle was found other anxieties needed my careful attention. Firstly, the hygienics of a toilet seat of a boy's school toilet, enough said there. Secondly whether there was enough toilet roll - not just enough for that visit, but for the rest of the day too. Every one of my pockets was stuffed to the brim with tissues, with extra reserves in my backpack just in case. I would press on my pockets to flatten them as much as possible to avoid people noticing - and was prepared for any questioning with the 'I have a cold coming' excuse ready.

Next there was the incognito problem, not just the fear of a person seeing me go in or out of a toilet more than once a day, but the desire to not bring attention to myself whilst I was in the cubicle. This only makes sense when you can appreciate that each visit was a minimum of five minutes (but could easily be 20 - 30 minutes), and that the sounds I produced were not exactly typical - the smell wasn't a major concern as this was usually masked by the existing climate. If someone came into the room it became a waiting game, the worst situation being when someone was waiting to use the cubicle after me. And finally, there was the trepidation of kids being kids; anyone in a cubicle is fair game. Kicking the door and banging on the rickety plastic walls, and even the practice of throwing sink water over the top was commonplace. It's safe to say I had other things on my mind than learning when at school. I didn't seek out help from the school, my teachers would know that I'd be in and out of class, but I kept most of these things to myself. I couldn't see how they (or anyone) could help, so my struggles remained my personal secret – all bottled up.

It could be said that I was my own worst enemy, as stress always makes things worse. It is hard to argue that my anxieties and rigorous routines weren't over the top, but this was the only way I knew. Advice like 'it is fine to prepare and plan, but don't let it control your life', and 'don't overthink it' didn't really hit home. As with any teenager, I needed to work this out in my own way. To teenagers their circumstance is unique, no-one else can fully understand. Chronic illness magnifies this, you feel more alone, more disconnected.

My treatment stepped-up to the more potent drug Infliximab*, and later Adalimumab*. For the most part, these granted me longer stretches of adequate health, allowing me to settle into some sort of routine. My fearful and overthinking state was ever-present, but I became more accustomed to the daily obstacles of the school week, with a trip to hospital for my next dose every other weekend.

There were still peaks and troughs in my health, a blood transfusion and short steroid courses were still sometimes unavoidable as well as other new medications introduced, such as Mesalazine granules and Prednisolone suppositories. One of the more poignant periods of these secondary school years was when we were forced into implementing a full liquid diet.

A low-fibre, low-residue liquid eases the strain on your bowels, helping your digestive system recover. The drink made by mixing a powder into water provides you with complete nutrition - which has benefits in itself. I'd had Modulen as a supplement to my diet before, but having the drink as every meal becomes harder over time.

It was good at the beginning, I felt better and the drink was still fresh, but a disdain for the taste and smell eventually starts to build up. There is no break from it, you have to consume a large volume each day, and are not allowed anything with it, no small plain biscuit or even a sip of juice.

Infliximab / Adalimumab – both are biological drugs that target a protein in the body (TNF-alpha). The protein is connected to the immune response; the goal is to suppress the immune system, which helps to control inflammation – but in turn this also decreases the body's ability to fight infection. Infliximab is given intravenously as an infusion, usually in hospital, over approximately 2 hours – you then are monitored for a further 2-3 hours in case of a reaction. Adalimumab is a painful subcutaneous injection (under the skin), this requires going into hospital initially - if you are a child - to receive it, but later you can receive deliveries of a pre-filled injection pen.

The only exception is a clear hardboiled sweet - two or three a day maximum.

At school it was something else I tried to hide, segregating myself at lunchtime. I didn't want to pull out the same flask every day in the dining hall, I was given access to a staff office where I could privately ingest the drink. After a few months on the strict diet my contempt for the drink was almost total. The technique I eventually adopted to force it down each meal was pouring it out into a cup, pinching my nose, and positioning a straw right to the back of my mouth - to avoid the tongue. After a few big gulps I would have a quick suck on the sweet I had already stuffed in my cheek. As you get through the thick liquid it feels heavier as it fills you up. By the time I had finished my attempt to get through the required volume, most of the lunch hour would be over. Towards the end of this treatment, as my motivation was nearly fully drained, I would simply give up after a few cups, abandon most of the drink and leave watery-eyed for the playground.

This is another thing I look back on and think, 'Why did you make such a fuss? Just down it, it is making you better!'... but perhaps it is easy to say this when you're not a hundred flasks deep. The benefits the diet brought weren't quite as miraculous as the steroids, but the improvements were swift and clear to see - with considerable weight gain and much more normal poos! But you can't stay on the diet forever, so finally we would ease back onto solid foods - I persuaded the doctor to push the schedule back a week so I was fully back onto a normal diet for Christmas dinner – a big win.

This was the first time a full liquid diet was prescribed to provide a respite for my bowels. A couple of years later after a short hospital stay and another colonoscopy it was decided it was required again.

It is known that returning to the diet is more difficult than the first time - as you know what is coming and already have built up negative ideas about the act of consuming it. We determined that a tube up my nose into the stomach was the best option, this is known as enteral feeding. This stays in - day and night - for the entire treatment period.

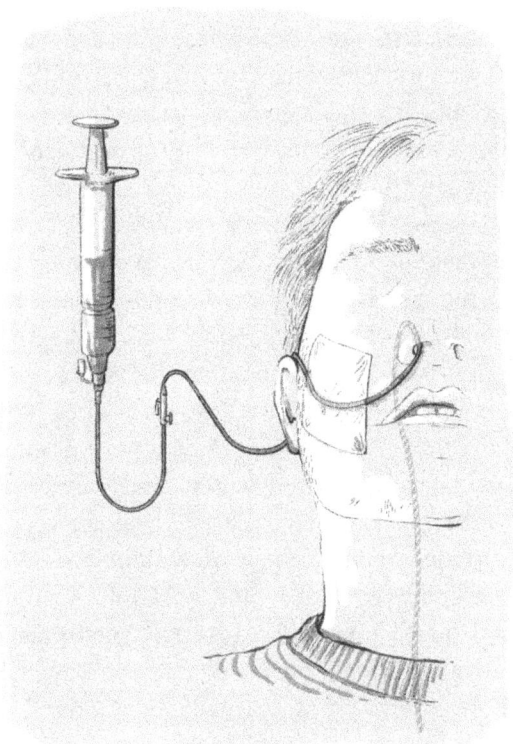

Putting the tube in isn't a nice experience. As it is slowly fed in, there is a strange pressure and scratching behind your nose and underneath the eye, as it bends down into the top of the throat. It tickles as it passes the back of the mouth - you are in limbo between retching and wanting to sneeze. On the first attempt the tube unfortunately bent in the throat, so had to be removed. After a little break the nurse tried again and was successful. Once it's in - other than when you swallow – you get used to the unusual feeling of something foreign dangling in your oesophagus and quickly forget about the part taped to your face.

Being fed or feeding yourself enterally is peculiar but not unpleasant. Each meal time you start by attaching a small syringe to the nose end of the tube and gently pull. This is to check that the other end is in the stomach and not the lungs - performing a pH test on the drawn-up liquid confirms this. Then the tube is flushed with water to ensure it is open and unclogged. Now we are ready for the feed. My mum premixed the solution each morning and stored it in the fridge. A large syringe filled with Modulen is then attached to the nose end and slowly pumped up. There is an enjoyable cold sensation in your nose and throat, and you feel your belly hastily expand, which feels a little odd when you aren't chewing or swallowing anything. In a very short period, you go from hungry to incredibly stuffed, it is only towards the end that it becomes uncomfortable, as you are very full but still need to squeeze down the last few syringes.

Again, this began to soothe the Crohn's within a few weeks, the tube allowing me to easily pump the correct volume. It didn't bother me, I'd rather have stayed tube fed than face the anxieties of school, but after an extended period

- once this deep relapse was tempered - the tube was removed and I returned to school.

Other than prolonged absences like this, it was only every so often that something would interfere with the daily routines I had designed - elevating the mental pressure above the school day norms. Simple things like a lesson with a replacement teacher signalled 'potential trouble ahead', when for other children it was a chance to misbehave and have a fun relaxing lesson.

The teacher did not know me or my toilet allowances - which could be up to five times in a one-hour lesson. A substitute teacher once told me 'you should have gone at break-time!' Absolutely hating attention being brought onto me going, I took a minute, but concluded that I couldn't hold off until the end of the class. So, I had to find the courage to confront her with my 'special IBD card' that stated *I have a condition necessitating urgent access to facilities.*

This put the teacher and I in an awkward and precarious situation; although she was just following the normal policies, on this occasion she was openly shown to be mistaken. I felt like I was inflicting a public shaming on her and myself. Besides this, for the remainder of the lesson (and any subsequent lessons I had with the same pupils) I'd be extremely anxious about going to the toilet again, as in my head everyone would definitely notice - looking to see if I had to use my card again.

Even more rudimentary things like cross-country P.E sessions added further unease. The far end of the circuit could be 15 minutes from the changing rooms toilet, although I probably set faster times because of this.

Perhaps the most unorthodox day, (certainly one of the most eventful days at school) involved me missing the opportunity to legitimately push a fire alarm button - let's face it we all wish we could do this once. I was in a lesson in one of my favoured quadrants of the campus; it was relatively small and set away from most of the school. Only servicing a smallish number of classrooms, the toilet block here was generally well kept. Typically, as with most of these stories, it begins with me needing the loo; indicating this to the teacher, he gave me a nod and I promptly left. I did my accelerated walk down the stairs to the toilet with my mind focused on the normal pains and clenching. I hurriedly push the door open and started my well-trodden beeline to the cubicles on the other side of the room. However, bizarrely, the room was dark and smelled different, I stepped back out confused. I re-entered and was still a bit befuddled, preoccupied with very much needing to be sat down in the cubicle. It didn't fully register that the room was filled with thick black smoke, I could barely see more than a metre forward – it really isn't something you expect to find! Upon noticing a glow from under one of the cubicles it became clear - the toilet roll dispenser had been set alight.

This was a predicament; needing to warn people about the fire, but also not pooing in my pants. I still really needed the toilet and the closest one was now further than expected, it was actually much further as the block that would be next nearest was closed for repairs that week. I had a split second to make a decision. If I set off the fire alarm, I would 100% be putting myself in a public soiling situation. The masses of people heading to the assembly point would be going against where I needed to go; there would be a full audience to my humiliation. They would prevent me getting there speedily and one person heading away from the assembly area would look very odd, any teacher would certainly stop me and ask what I was doing - I didn't have time for that. On the other hand, there was a fire, although it wasn't a raging inferno, there was still a lot of smoke.

I ran to the classroom next to the toilet, interrupted the class in session with 'erm... there's a fire... you should probably get out.' I then went back upstairs to the room above the toilet and did the same, and then to my classroom one along from this. I then sprinted to the toilets that weren't on fire... made it! After a while I headed to the fire assembly point, the alarm hadn't been raised, only the quadrant in question had been evacuated. There was a nod and smile with my teacher as I saw him realise the muddle I had just stumbled into. The fire department came and a boy was excluded.

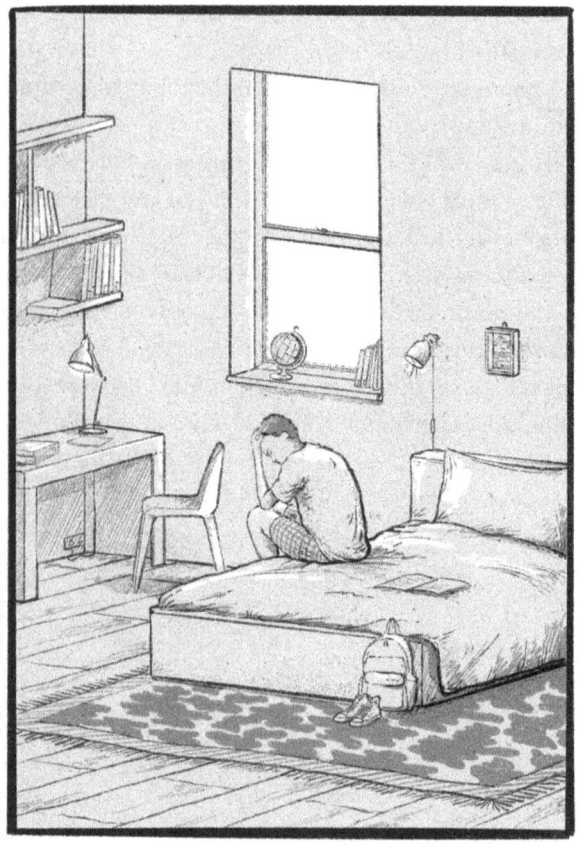

- The Crohn Ranger -

I have spoken primarily about how the disease affected me or disrupted my school day in terms of logistics and tactics; I will now move on to how it affected my relationships, and ability to connect with people.

I wasn't a recluse or lonely during school hours, and was on friendly terms with almost everyone in my year, but it was difficult to maintain a close or 'best' friendship for more than a year. I believe an amalgamation of factors contributed to this.

I missed a lot of school, but not as much as you may expect. I went in most days and if things got bad, I could always be picked up. Though, when I was in the classroom or around my friends at break times, I wasn't fully 'there' most of the time. In any public situation a significant portion of my mind was somewhere else, incessantly running risk analysis on the best time to eat, the quickest route to the toilets, what would I do if I used up the masses of toilet tissue I had in every pocket (a sock was my finest proposition), focusing on any tummy twinges that might give me some warning, and also worrying if people noticed these things. I do not know if this disengagement was obvious to others, but it definitely played a role from my end. I inadvertently kept myself at a distance by presenting a restrained, dispassionate version of myself. I probably came across as disinterested and moody - either uninvolved in the conversation or bitter for an unknown reason.

Whether consciously or not I also detached myself in another way; by confining my friendships to within the school gates. This was the age where you start to hang-out without parents - meeting up on weekends, going to the cinema, parties. All of which I avoided. This withdrawal from 'normal social activities' understandably acted as a barricade, as most couldn't relate as to why. Furthermore, I didn't want to explain myself, as I felt it would be awkward or seen as silly that the justification was that 'I can't come because I don't know if there is a toilet there.' Giving the real reason would have meant openly discussing my illness, something that I was not ready to do. After a while people stop inviting you. This is not a criticism, at all. I built the barriers and couldn't expect people to break through them. The person they met was blurred and darkened, obscured by a hidden disease.

Maybe I wasn't brave enough, I shouldn't have worried or cared as much, but from my viewpoint the risks were high and appeared to heavily outweigh the positives. There is a self-imposed shame, facing the stigma is a big step. A judgemental, ridicule ridden school environment is not the easiest place to reach the milestone of accepting and 'owning' the illness. I was still a few years away from building up the self-confidence to be fully forthcoming about myself and my condition. There may be a shift in respectfulness and accepting people's differences and needs in society nowadays, but I suspect this will take a longer time to filter down into schools, where trivial things like wearing glasses or hair colour are enough to be taunted.

It wasn't like this from the start, I participated in many sports and tried to get out of the house when I felt up to it, but slowly my confidence and motivation was chipped away by my self-isolation from friends and by some indecent incidents.

These provided excuses, to myself, to be more protective and remain in my safety bubble.

A key example of this started with a friend staying over at mine, with plans to play tennis the following day - we were around 14-years-old. I wasn't in a deep relapse or in remission, and knew the tennis club quite well - the courts were near the clubhouse and the toilets were in a good condition, so I was content with adventuring out. I did my normal pre-leaving the house risk-reduction procedures, but with the added masquerade for my friend. Avoiding eating was 'I don't know, I'm just not hungry today', and showering, brushing my teeth and blowing my nose were all ways to give myself a few extra minutes in the bathroom straining on the toilet.

We weren't playing long before I had to pop to the loo, I would always say 'I need to take a leak' or 'have a wee', it seemed less embarrassing than pooing. In a situation like this where someone is waiting for me, it always felt like there was a floodlight and stop clock on me going to the toilet. I would rush there, push and push, wipe, clean my hands and rush back; not wanting my friend to be left alone too long and start to wonder what I was doing. After a few minutes I had to go again. Laughing it off, 'I probably didn't finish last time, there's a bit left'. Hurriedly again, I tensed and strained, not much in the bowl, but the pain had gone and there were no more movements inside, so hastily I headed back out to the court. Five minutes later, that feeling again. I couldn't leave the court for a third time in under 15 minutes! It felt like it could just be a fart, so between points I took the chance. Let's just say I wasn't fit to continue.

I remember it so distinctly because of the charming phone conversation with my step-dad. 'Hi, Mike'... 'Hi Kev...can you pick us up, I've shit myself'.

It's not something you really get used to, standing there in soggy pants with poo running down your leg. Panic and focussing on the next move usually overcame the shame, all I could do was smile and try to make light of it. Having a sense of humour is generally the best way to handle Crohn's (sometimes the only way) but this can be much easier said than done. The friend was aware I had an illness, and was understanding. As we waited to be picked up, using the tennis racket case to cover myself, I joked that 'I was going to 'get it' at school next week.' We laughed and he said not to worry. To be fair it was not spread around the school, I only heard one comment he made to another friend. 'Why is he walking like that...it's like he has shat himself.'

At school people knew I wasn't well from all my absences, but I didn't give any real details unless circumstance 'forced' me to. For instance, it was made very clear to my tennis companion without me having to verbally explain it. Another such instance is when I invited a new friend over after school. On the walk home from the bus stop, I suddenly very urgently had to go. Without time to explain, I said 'Sorry, but I really have to go... can you hold this?!' I dumped my backpack and gym bag on him and sprinted around the corner. For him, this was a bit strange I'm sure, especially since he didn't know which house or even which street was mine. From his perspective I had randomly run away from him, leaving him in the middle of an unknown area, with two extra bags.

Typically, I didn't make it home in time. As I hurried to the shower, I shouted to my mum to go out and find my friend 'He doesn't know where the house is!' This incident clearly required some explanation; when I was decent again, I laughed it off and told him only what I felt I had to - a minimal explanation. The same way I didn't risk trusting my bowels enough to leave the house when not necessary, I didn't risk trusting people to tell them unless I really had to.

My sports and social activities slowly all dropped away; tennis, table-tennis, diving, swimming and obviously cricket - wearing all white in an open field for hours on end was really pushing my luck flirting with a code brown situation. Even football was too difficult to continue, the stress of home matches was ample, but travelling away to unknown fields proved too much. The worry stopped me eating any breakfast and lunch before a game each Saturday. The added difficulty is that in team sports, you can't just slip away to the loo, your teammates are depending on you.

Away from school, my life became very deprived of social interaction (other than family). Always at home and lonely, I gravitated to the social engagement online computer games offered. It did not matter that I didn't really know the friends I made through the microphone. It was a social outlet I could happily participate in whilst feeling safe. They couldn't see I was ill, and I could just enjoy chatting about nothing and play mindlessly, without worries.

It did develop into a bit of an obsession - playing until the early hours most weekends. With so much free time I ended up becoming top ten in the world for one game; probably not the most advisable hobby for kids, but it was making me happy and it wasn't like I had any reason to get up early. Many hours were 'wasted' on those games, but it was my escape, my coping mechanism. Retreating into a different world is something everyone can relate to; some might read or exercise or watch films, a break from their norm. It was a great distraction for me through tough times.

With no desire to make any plans for any evening or any weekend, my mid-teenage years all merge together. Securely stuck in my play-it-safe mentality and life. During these years of home - school - home - hospital - home I of course felt like I was missing out, and my isolation created some resentment towards others. My classmates were enjoying themselves, meeting up, meeting girls, but I had other priorities. I tried not to let this overly frustrate me, it was the life I knew and just continued to plod through it. This sounds quite depressing I know, there are happy memories from this time, but my overwhelming image of my adolescence is feeling rubbish, trapped and lonely. On reflection, I do feel robbed of that time. Now I try to make up for this 'lost time', making the best of good health.

It wasn't just my friendships that were affected, my family relationships were also under strain. The key factor in this was my mood. I always had this anger bubbling underneath; angry at everything and everyone for reasons I did not fully understand. I was irritable and on the edge of a bad mood for almost a decade. This may have just been the normal teenage experience, but I don't think it was just that. The disease and the medication play havoc with your system and therefore mood. But, even knowing these contributing factors it still grinds everyone down eventually, especially the people you spend every day with. I spent the most time with my mum, not just the more than usual time at home, when I couldn't go to school - sometimes for weeks on end, but she also accompanied me to every hospital appointment, and commuted in to be with me every day I was on the ward. What an effort it must have been to tolerate me in that state for such a long time.

The extent of the strain and pressures on my parents and family life in general is probably best told from my parents' perspective. This will be recounted in chapter 'Parental Guidance', but let's stay with my own experience of the disease for now.

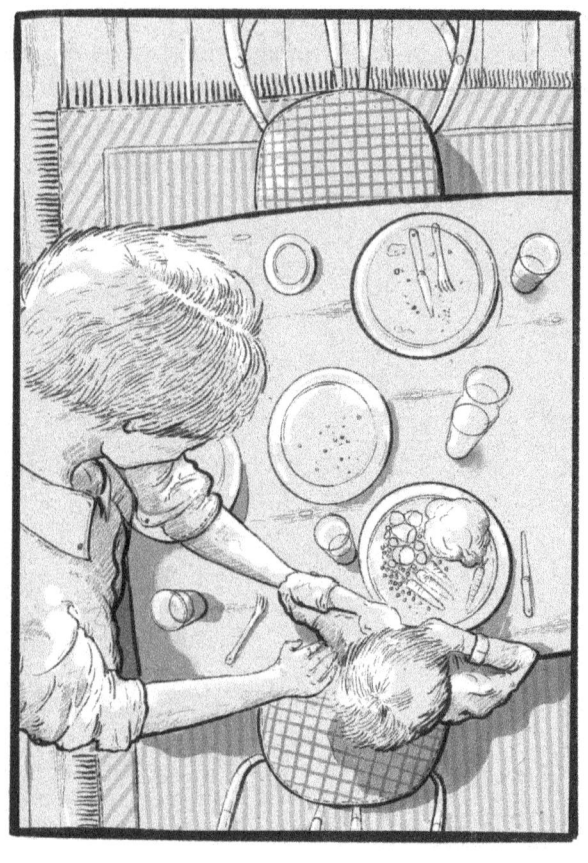

- FOOD FIGHT!!! -

Dinner times were the catalyst for many arguments at home, my fussy eating being the central topic. My parents, the doctors (and I'm sure my body) wanted me to eat well; a varied and sufficient diet, not just to gain weight and grow, but also to overcome a diseased gut's inefficient nutrition absorption. Opposing this was my robust fear of food, more specifically new foods. Each day it was a 'normal' meal for everyone else, and a separate plainer version for me.

Eating enough was a secondary issue, it was the lack of variety that really frustrated my parents. I had a very stripped-down diet; I didn't want to try anything that I hadn't eaten before. This started because of the fear of the unknown, a different meal or even a single new vegetable was terrifying - as I didn't know how it would make me feel afterwards. This cemented itself over time, I became more and more stubborn and strict about sticking only to my tried and tested foods - in the end forgetting the real reason I didn't want to try and just knowing not to.

Eating was a chore, purely for sustenance. Food didn't bring pleasure only the possibility of pain; it wasn't until my mid to late twenties that I really started to expand my diet and be more open to new things. There are still foods that I just won't even consider, but these generally align with things I probably should avoid anyway - namely things that are too spicy, too saucy or too greasy.

This wasn't a mild phobia; I didn't like the look, I didn't like the smell, just the thought of something unfamiliar (even ketchup or gravy!) near my food struck genuine dread in me.

There wasn't much logic to it either, and it wasn't just about 'good' foods, i.e. me trying to avoid my vegetables. A typical example - one that would really aggravate my parents - was jam doughnuts, I would eat plain ringed doughnuts and would eat jam tarts, but I wouldn't touch a jam doughnut or jam by itself. Go figure.

A few things were tried to overcome this mental block. One was to introduce a new simple food, like rice, once a week or so. I would agree in principle, but when it was actually there on the plate, I was paralysed to even touch it with my fork. I would pick around it, try to hide it, anything to avoid eating it. Sometimes I would be at the table for nearly two hours waiting for my parents to give up for the evening.

Another (picked up by my parents from scouring the internet I'm sure) was an attempt to de-demonise the food, by touching it. The idea is to make a connection with the food, without an intent or any pressure on it going anywhere near my mouth. An unliked food is placed on a plate and you use your hand to push it around - hopefully realising that it isn't this toxic horrible substance that I had built it up to be. It was proposed that it would be mashed potato with ketchup on it, again, I agreed thinking it would be easy - I'm not eating it right? But again, when it came to it I couldn't. I was in tears as I pulled my hand away as my step-dad pushed it to simply touch the food. This is quite a funny image to me now, but clearly the phobia was very well ingrained.

It wasn't just my parents; my grandma once tried a more creative approach, which she didn't really think through. Cutting open some homemade meatballs revealed small bits of spaghetti that had been concealed within. With a limited diet, my palate was always going to detect something alien, and furthermore - although I understand the eagerness for me to eat better - I now hold this loving betrayal accountable as to why I won't eat any type of pasta today.

My parents even went to the extreme of taking me to a hypnotist. To clarify, I did want to eat better and was open to these experiments but there was this barrier - that I am struggling to fully explain (or even understand) - preventing me from making any progress. We arrived at a suburban house and entered a large, peaceful lounge. With my parents sitting to the side of the room, the hypnotherapist ran through some IQ test questions and then lightly questioned me about my diet. Then it was time for the main event. I was told to relax my body, concentrate on my breathing, feel myself becoming sleepy (all as the movies tell us), but all I could think was that I really needed to scratch my nose. I held off for a good 5 minutes, while the therapist softly tried to 'put me under', but eventually I had to do it. Slowly (in an attempt to stay in a soothed state) I raised my hand to scratch my nose. It was suddenly very hard to stay tranquil as I could hear my parents trying to hold back the giggles - I guess the sight of me laying back and slowly lifting my arm was too much. We persisted for the rest of the session, but there was no going back - we still laugh about this today. This bizarre experience didn't seem like such an eccentric step at the time, it was just another treatment or test. It shows the desperation my parents had for me to eat.

At this time, I was rarely in a situation where my diet was awkward for me, or open to external pressures from outside of the family - such as from friends. This is mainly because I didn't get out much, but also as there wasn't the massive food culture of today; I can imagine it would be difficult now with the thousands of self-proclaimed nutritionists telling everyone what they *must* eat. Diet wasn't raised as an issue by the doctors - other than to be careful with the amount of fibre; I did have meetings with dietitians, but the advice and goals set were always about calories and getting the vitamins – no mention of obscure herbs or ground seeds.

In adulthood there has been improvement, I have a better attitude towards food and my diet has grown. It has mainly expanded along similar lines; as in within the same food 'types' - with a wider variety of meat and fish, fruit and vegetables. Still no stews, or soups…or pasta. In the last few years, some things I actively hated the sight of are now staple foods, such as eggs and fish, I even tried mussels a few weeks ago! Diluting the phobia was a gradual thing, it wasn't a case of becoming bored of the same foods, more that I became bored of the fears - in most cases anyway. Not outgrowing them, outliving them.

My girlfriend is a foodie, which also has definitely played a part. She has a good way of encouraging without there being any pressure; cooking something plain on the side - separate from our meal - for me to try a small piece if I felt like it. Or using a blender to add a new fruit or something like spinach to a smoothie - so that the act of trying it isn't direct, but I can see that it isn't horrendous and can slowly become familiar to the new taste, and in time eat it in its natural state. These methods aren't dissimilar to what my parents were trying to do, but now post-surgery with a better outlook on life, food and well everything, I am more open to change.

The main obstacle left is when we eat out, primarily when we are invited to eat out (when we can't select a restaurant that satisfies her 'foodiness', but also has a few simpler options for me); it requires menu research. What I try to avoid is ordering something and having to say to the waiter 'can I have this, but WITHOUT this and this'. No one likes their issues or insecurities being publicised.

There is still progress to be made, sauces are still my nemesis and there is still 'the fear' when I see something unexpected on the plate, but we will get there… eventually.

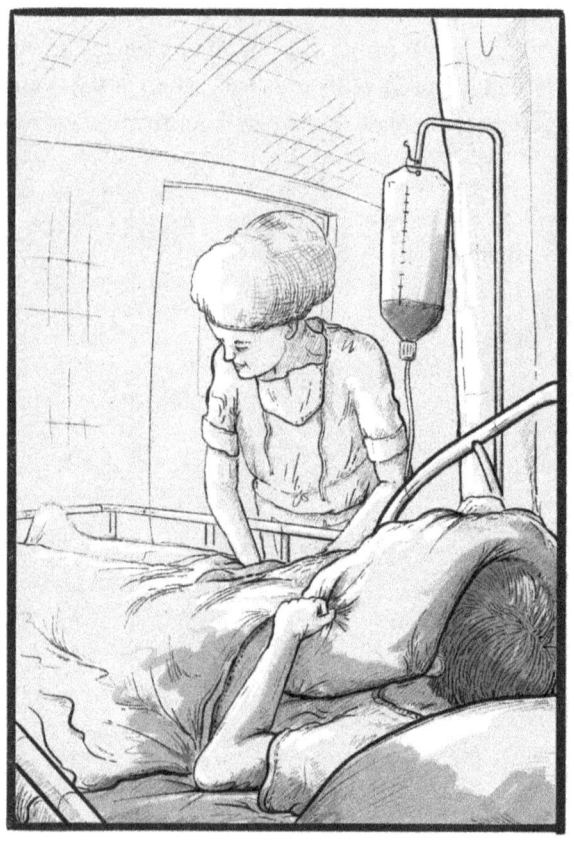

- Gut Outta Here -

Secondary school was coming to an end, so it was time for the final (GCSE) exams. The added pressures from exams would make my symptoms worse, which would make me more concerned about sitting in a quiet hall, for up to three hours at a time... which in turn would then make my health (and state of mind) deteriorate further - a vicious spiral. Even with my IBD card, and a teacher arranging for me to sit near the front door of the hall (closer to the toilets), I would still worry more about my toilet needs than the actual tests themselves. I worried about needing multiple toilet visits and therefore not finishing the questions, and even thought the invigilators would query the amount of time I took, accuse me of cheating and prevent me from going again.

My school was one with a college attached (sixth form), and thankfully I did well enough in my GCSE exams to allow me to stay there to study A-Levels. Over that summer and the first few months of college, my health became completely out of control. In and out of hospital or housebound, I missed a lot of days and was in a bad way when at school; almost completely withdrawn into myself, surrounded by the Crohn's.

All available drugs had been exhausted; double, triple and quadruple doses couldn't bring me out of relapse. A permanent fully liquid diet or more steroids were not sustainable long-term solutions, they would have only been further delaying the inevitable - cutting out the disease.

I had heard the words 'having a bag' before, but they always ignited great fear inside of me. I refused to even discuss it - even a mention made me instantly tearful, angry, and full of terror. Most people do not have any real idea of what an ostomy bag looks like, where it goes, what it is for, or how it works. I was the same - I had this image in my head of a supermarket plastic carrier bag taped to me. The fear not only stemmed from the unknown, but also from the misconceptions that bags are dirty, smelly and only meant for old people.

Being healthy didn't enter my mind. I thought that getting a bag was the end of hope for any normal life in the future; I would be more different and have another thing to hide and be embarrassed (even ashamed) about. Who would want to be friends with or want to date someone with literally a bag of shit hanging off them? Even though I had developed a good mask to hide behind, I was already in a hole of insecurity, adding body image issues to this was going to make this even deeper.

I sat in silence twiddling my thumbs as the consultant told my mum there aren't any real options other than surgery. I only remember that sentence and my mum turning to me and saying 'Come on Mikey, it's time'.

Was I going to have loads of scars? Was there literally going to be a hole in me? How big, where? How, when, where is it cleaned, or even if it is? Who does it? Am I going to smell? There were so many questions that I did not want to ask, and did not want to know the answers to. Asking would make it real.

Things moved very fast, within a day a stoma nurse was explaining the procedure and showing us various bags, wipes, adhesives and other ostomy bag 'equipment'. I didn't want to listen and learn; I was still digesting the news.

That day or the next, I was on a drip in my hospital bed when the surgical team came to talk to us. The head surgeon said I was booked in for after the weekend, but 'luckily' he could rejig a few things and fit me in tomorrow. I had chosen to ignore the news, distracting myself from it, so a doctor telling me he could remove my bowel tomorrow... well, I certainly wasn't ready for that. We kept the original slot so I could go home, collect my thoughts and enjoy what I thought was my last few days of 'normality', with my life going downhill from here. There was also a final hope that things could change over the weekend and I wouldn't need the surgery.

I continued to avoid thinking about what I thought was my impending doom until the night before I was going back into hospital. It was hard to know what aspect to worry about or fear the most; a life pooing into a bag, people's perceptions of this, or the actual surgery itself. I was in my room crying at 3am (very out of character), the surgery was inescapable now, I was trapped by it, there was nowhere to hide, this thing I had feared for years was now on my doorstep. My mum heard and came in, I didn't have to explain, she knew everything I was distressed about and knew I couldn't see the wider picture - that this was a chance for a better life, not the opposite. We read through the leaflets on the surgery, on what to expect after and got the sample bag 'equipment' out. It all looked so odd, these odd shapes with weird opening mechanisms - we filled a bag up with water in an attempt to understand it better. The bag looked so big held against my thin, meagre body. It was going to be so obvious, sticking out so much from my scrawny frame. It didn't really matter that consoling words like 'plenty of people have it, have you ever noticed it on anyone?' did not comfort me, as like I said there were no other options now.

My hospital was one of few in the UK with a special adolescent ward (11-16 year-olds). Even though I was 17 they decided I was best placed here - rather than in an adult ward. My body wasn't an adult body, so a paediatric surgeon was deemed more suitable. I was thankful for this as to me an adult ward meant the real world, scary, big and different; a place I was not ready for. I belonged in my room, on my toilet; my world was small and insular.

I remember arriving in the familiar ward, opening the door and seeing Laura - my favourite nurse - she was always upbeat, cheery and smiley (and I may have had a little crush on her…). I didn't know what she was doing, but she stood in the hallway with a wide plastic apron on, gloves and a large face-shielding visor on her head. She spotted my mum and me, threw her hand in the air and loudly welcomed us. The funny sight made me instantly feel much more relaxed, and I wasn't able to hold back a smile - a rare occurrence that week. The only other thing I really recall about the day and night before the surgery was that I stayed up into the early hours talking to the night-shift nurses - holding onto my last day and wanting to avoid upsetting myself by thinking about tomorrow.

I am so thankful for all the staff - the National Health Service here in the UK is the most amazing thing. I remember and thank the nurses, the doctors, and the cleaner whom I chatted to everyday. I always defend and speak up when I hear any bad word about the NHS - anyone moaning about having to wait 40 minutes for a blood test just has no idea.

My procedure was an ileostomy with a sub-total colectomy. In short, my large colon (where my disease was most active) was removed, with a small piece (a rectal stump) left at the anus end - where the bowel could potentially be reconnected one day. This left me with a thin scar about 7 inches long (cutting vertically through my belly button) and a stoma. A stoma is the piece of bowel brought out through the abdomen - it looks like a little red strawberry stuck onto the skin. As it is a piece of bowel it sometimes moves (a little bit) by itself, and grows and shrinks slightly. An ostomy bag (sometimes called an appliance or pouch) goes over and around the strawberry, sticking to the surrounding skin. My digestive system is basically missing the last section, and instead of my waste going out of my bottom, it now exits through the stoma into a bag… and then to a toilet.

I woke up with a large array of tubes and new things entering or coming out of me. A total of eight if you include the stoma. In case you're interested - two cannulas (both hands), a morphine line, a weird upper arm/shoulder needle, a catheter, an epidural (spine), and an enteral (nose) feeding tube.

As my grogginess started to wear off, thoughts that 'it was done' drifted in and out, I was still in denial. I didn't want to open my eyes or speak. But I couldn't ignore a pain that slowly started to emanate from the top of my belly just below the chest. It was just uncomfortable at first but over a couple of hours the pain spread slowly down, the further it went the more intense it was. Conversely my legs were totally and completely numb, I couldn't move them or feel any sensation. My epidural was checked but it seemed to be fine from the outside; something wasn't though, as clicking the morphine button as soon as it let me wasn't holding the pain back (morphine drips are on a timer to prevent overdose - after a certain amount of time you can click the button to get some more). This was not normal Crohn's pain, it was a hot, deep, pulsing burn emanating from the lower part of my tummy - where I had been cut open and rearranged. The 'pain team' were called as my discomfort became very clear to see. On a scale of 1-10, I graded the pain an 11. Within a couple of minutes, I was given a larger dose of something (I assumed morphine) and was out like a light.

My legs were completely numb for at least another day - the spinal epidural hadn't done its job quite right. It is supposed to numb you from the belly down, mine just skipped the belly part. Over the next few days, I was still very sore with regular pain medication keeping things at bay for the most part. The most painful thing I have ever experienced is retching post-surgery. There is no eating for a while so it was only bile (or nothing) that I was bringing up. I have a high pain threshold but seriously, wow, the intensity when my freshly reorganised insides tensed to throw-up, no words. The funny thing was that the anti-nausea meds that I would get every few hours would consistently make me heave 10-15 minutes later, even if I was asleep when it was administered - fortunately we realised this pattern and stopped these after a couple of days.

I lay in the half sat-up position with a pillow over my stomach area. The catheter was new but I could also feel something else foreign - the bag and stoma within. I couldn't bring myself to look down, or touch anywhere near it. When the nurse came to empty or change the bag, I could smell it. I'd turn my head, grit my teeth and close my eyes as the nurse rubbed and rustled around, I didn't know what she was doing but it didn't feel good, the area was raw and tender. When it was done, I promptly returned the pillow, it was my shield, I couldn't face whatever was down there.

I still tried my best not to the think about the stoma, distract myself in any way so as not to picture the monstrosity I'd been imagining.

My mum came every day and other family members every so often, I didn't say much but was very glad for the interruption from my own thoughts. Another massive thank you to my mum, for just being by my bed and understanding why and when I needed to be encouraged or left alone - it would have been much harder without you! The same goes to the nurses and doctors who, as always, were also amazing.

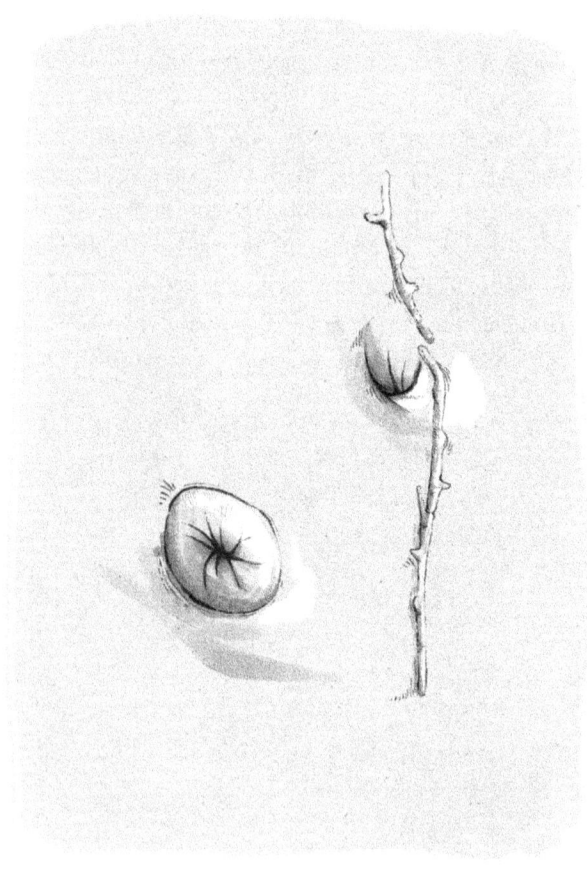

- Ileostomy, Myself and I -

After about eight days the throwing-up had fully subsided and the stitches (central scar and around the stoma) were healing well. It was time for the catheter to come out, not the nicest feeling this one, but what it meant was worse; I would now have to go to the bathroom to urinate and therefore be alone with the bag for the first time.

Whether it was the first visit or not, I soon decided to have my first peak in the mirror. Firstly I moved the gown to reveal the scar, it looked pretty badass to be honest, and then after a minute or so I unveiled the main event. First impressions... weren't great. It wasn't the supermarket bag I had previously imagined, but it still looked so big and alien. It could have been half the size and pretty and I still wouldn't have been happy. It was an alarming, undesirable change to my body, I was never going to be happy with it. It took weeks, even months before I became used to it, much longer before I was conformable with other people knowing, and even longer before fully understanding myself the real value it brought to my life.

Most appliances (bags) have this skin-coloured material over the actual watertight plastic pouch (to conceal the contents), it took a few more trips before I was ready to pull this aside to see the stoma itself. It is such a peculiar, interesting sight, this small blob of insides stitched onto the outside, but again, you get used to seeing and touching (when cleaning and changing) this too. To be discharged I had to demonstrate to my stoma nurse that I could independently deal with my new passenger. Now it's like tying my shoe, but initially there was a lot of new information to digest.

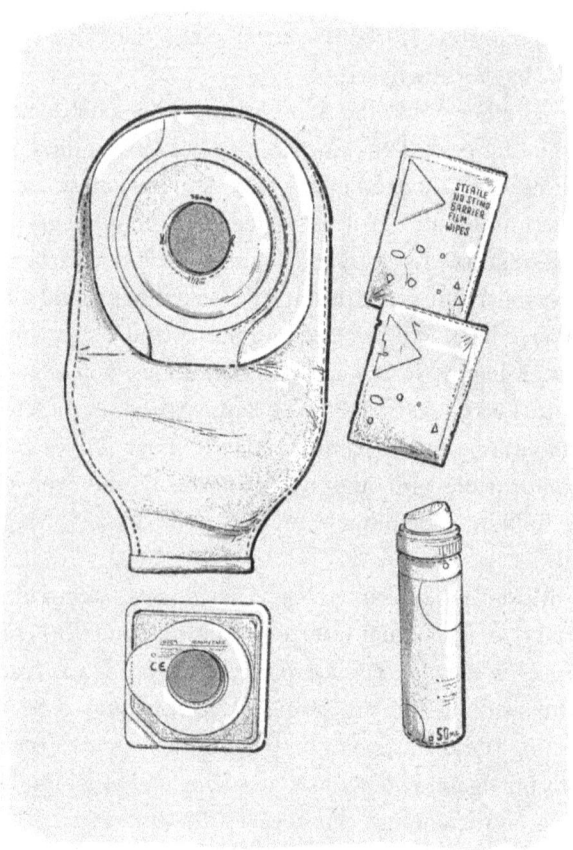

There are many types of ileostomy pouches from multiple manufacturers. The most common drainable types are one-piece (which I use) and two-piece systems. A typical one-piece is a plastic water-tight pouch, with an emptying mechanism at the bottom. On the upper side, there is an adhesive 'plate'; a hole is cut into the centre of the plate (to the correct diameter) and this goes over the stoma. A two-piece system has a baseplate (adhesive flange surrounding the stoma) as an independent part - which bags are attached to (as opposed to attaching directly onto the skin). With this system the baseplate can stay in place for a few days with the attachable secondary bag being changed more often.

Bags are emptied (when they fill up throughout the day) into the toilet via the mechanism; with ileostomies the output is looser than conventional bowel movements, so emptying is gravity assisted and very straightforward – taking less than a minute. A bag change takes a little longer, requiring more than just toilet roll. The two-piece may differ slightly, but for a one-piece the process normally takes five minutes (but allow 10 minutes in case of hitches - like the stoma becoming active mid change). There are many slight divergences from this method - such as wipes instead of sprays, or wet versus dry wipes - but this is mine.

Whilst standing in front of the toilet a medical adhesive removing spray helps bring one of the top corners of the 'adhesive plate' away from the skin, whilst gently pulling at the detaching corner I spray a little more to encourage the whole plate (and therefore the bag) to completely be removed - this is then placed into a disposable bag. This is pain free other than maybe a few hairs being pulled out. We now have an exposed stoma that will likely be a little dirty (as well as some of the close surrounding skin at its base). I use a tap to wet some dry wipes and lightly clean the stoma and skin; removing any poo and adhesive left behind (there can be a very small amount of blood from the base of the stoma - where it is tied to the skin - but this is completely normal). Once clean and dabbed dry, using a skin friendly 'barrier film' wipe I wipe the whole area of skin that the bag's adhesive plate comes into contact with; offering protection to the skin, priming it for the next bag and any irritating faecal matter that may touch it. This dries quickly and now the site is ready for the next pouch; as an extra protection I first place a tacky 'barrier ring' directly around the stoma helping to seal the vulnerable area between the stoma's base and the bag - where poo may try to get under the adhesive plate. The pre-cut hole in the bag's plate goes over the stoma and onto the skin, after some pressing to ensure it is stuck all over you're ready to go.

It took about a year until I found a bag that was right for me. The brand I was initially provided with didn't 'agree' with me. I would have to change my bag two or three times a day, and have some close calls of it nearly leaking or partially coming off during the night. The faecal matter (as it can be basically liquid) was 'eating away' at the adhesive material surrounding the stoma, which then irritates the skin making it hard for the next bag to stick to. I didn't realise that this was avoidable and uncommon; once I raised the issue with a stoma nurse - she wasn't pleased that I had been having to change my bag at school - we trialled a few different bags and additional sticky elements (the barrier ring I mentioned earlier) and now I use one that isn't itchy and doesn't bring any risk of leaking for about two to three days, although I still choose to keep it fresh and change mine most days to limit my skin's contact with irritants.

Apologies if this summary is a little dry, but hopefully now you have a better understanding of what a bag really is and some of the maintenance required.

About two weeks after surgery I was deemed well enough to go home. The pain had settled, the scar was healing well, the rest of the tubes were removed - like plucking a porcupine - and I had shown I could competently empty and change my bag unassisted.

- A New Life? -

We met with my school, and it was decided that - with all the days I had already missed throughout the first half of the year and the couple of months around the surgery - I'd have to repeat the year.

I wasn't over the moon with this, I'd stand out as the new kid, there would be questions as to why I was in that year group, and I feared isolation at break times as I wouldn't know anyone - but it was clearly the only way. I told myself 'I'm used to this now', I can do a couple more years of being alone, get through this and I'll make friends at university or at work. This gave me six months, the plan being: fully recover, get more accustomed to bag-life, and make a start on building some self-confidence. This was a slow drawn-out process.

For weeks I still spent most of my time locked away in my room, not wanting to see people and refusing to discuss the surgery, the bag or anything about myself really. I had even more time on my hands without school and also with much fewer trips to the toilet! Spending hours on the loo each day is a pattern I have not totally left behind. To this day I still have 'phantom poos', much to my friends' amusement. I get the urge to sit on the toilet and push. About once a month I will just go and sit there for 10 minutes - obviously nothing happening - being so accustomed to that position and feeling, it's like an itch I just need to scratch.

Adapting to the bag procedures went smoothly, the stoma nurse only having to visit once or twice to check we were coping with the transition. Over time, I stopped protecting the stoma site with my hand, and in small bursts began to talk to the family about it. We gathered information and discussed the options available to me; what hobbies are suitable (perhaps not rugby), what I should take with me when leaving the house, and what accessories there are for comfort and concealing. For example, the bag's outline can be seen if just wearing a t-shirt - especially if it has some air in it, we found an 'ostomy elastic waistband' product that covers the whole belly area - gently holding the bag to my skin. I also researched (by myself) how having a bag affected relationships and sought advice for the more intimate activities. Again, gradually, I also began showing a select few family members the bag, and the stoma within.

Alongside this I began to realise I could do more, and importantly wanted to. I was much more comfortable away from the toilet, I still wanted to know there was one somewhat nearby (because the bag would still need emptying) but there was a considerably greater window of opportunity. Before my daily experience was waiting for the next pain or toilet urge, relief afterwards and then expecting, worrying and anticipating when it would come again. Everything else was just a distraction, a divergence from this primary routine. Now it was reversed, this was the second or third thought! Still present but not driving my actions. I could watch my football team, with my mind actually on the football! Not planning my bowel movements for the journey home! It was bizarre, I had forgotten what being healthy felt like.

With the worst of my disease removed, my appetite grew, there was no sprinting to the loo, no vomiting, no real pain, only a plastic thing on my belly that sometimes made one or two farting noises. My parent's words 'your life can really start now' began to make sense. I wouldn't say I was suddenly all optimistic and happy, but now feeling a 1000% better, with a head free from so many of the grinding incessant worries, my outlook improved. The end of this chapter was in sight, I thought Crohn's was now behind me.

A New Life?

The surgery had certified the diagnosis as Crohn's Disease - not Ulcerative Colitis. This potentially wasn't good news, as the removal of the large colon would have brought an end to Ulcerative Colitis, but as Crohn's reaches further, there was still a possibility it could continue to be active in other areas of the digestive tract.

Three months post-surgery, a few mild signs of the disease started to surface. Not a relapse at all, just a little blood from my back passage and some inflammation markers. Diversion Colitis occurs in the 'left-over' part of the bowel after surgery. It is said that the redundant pieces become irritated as they are no longer processing stools. This is a common post-ileostomy development; suppositories and enemas were quickly introduced to my ongoing medication. At this time, I had still thought or hoped that the stoma wasn't totally permanent, but was informed that with the Diversion Colitis, a reversal would not be possible - at least for the foreseeable future - the doctor even spoke about removing the final section (permanently erasing any chance of a reversal). I was a little taken back by this, but I was starting to realise the freedom I had been granted so it wasn't upsetting.

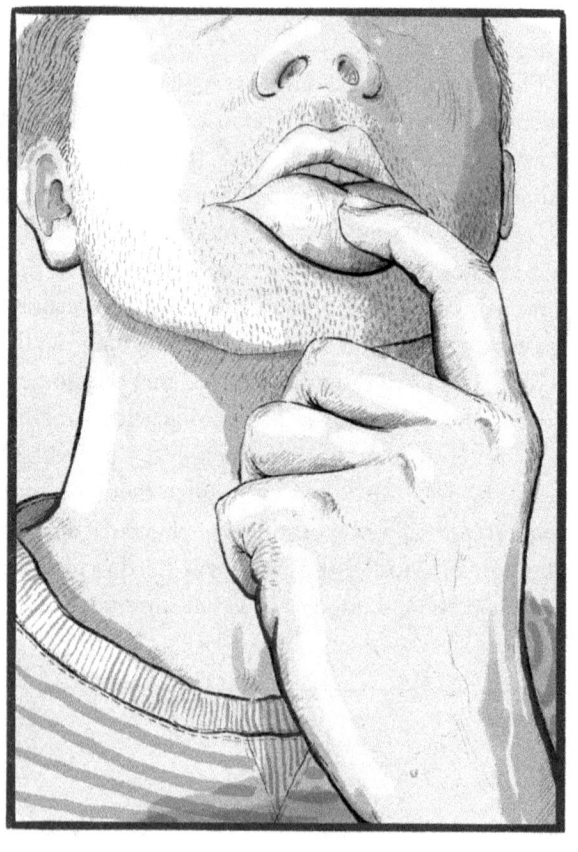

About two months before returning to school, the disease came back into my life in a far more uncommon way. After a summery day of family, food and football in the garden, I suddenly felt very tired in the early evening, so went to bed. Waking up a few hours later, around ten o'clock, I was sweating, feeling a little delirious and my mouth was sore. Half asleep I could feel my bottom lip was a bit swollen but nothing to worry about, I popped to the toilet and returned to bed. My mum hearing this, came to check I was okay "OH MY GOD, YOUR LIP!!! WHAT HAPPENED!??" I thought she was being a mum and over reacting... until I looked in the mirror.

The bottom half of my face, mainly my cheeks and bottom lip were inflamed to a ridiculous extent. I couldn't talk or swallow properly – the inside of my cheeks touching the sides of my tongue. We were very confused, had a bee stung me? Was it a reaction to a thorn or something from the garden? A couple of anti-histamines and ibuprofen, and surely it would go down soon. When it didn't, we went to the local hospital (not my IBD hospital). The A&E desk were a little taken aback by my lip and as there was a slight rash around it, I was pushed forward in the queue to see a doctor. They did the normal checks, on glands etc, and then sent me for a type of ultrasound to see what was going on under the surface of the lip. No one was sure what to make of it, we hadn't made the connection to Crohn's as it seemed so targeted to the lip. Maybe a food reaction? Maybe a reaction to my newly put in braces? We had them taken out... still no reduction in the swelling.

We had eliminated the obvious potential causes of the swelling and when it was clear it wasn't going to go away by itself, my IBD consultant referred me to another hospital that specialises in oral medicine as well as IBD. It was determined that it was Orofacial Granulomatosis (OFG) - thought to be a subtype of Crohn's. It manifests in a similar way with ulcers and inflammation but in the mouth area; it can result in permanent disfigurement of the lips and face. No longer able to operate in my large colon, my disease chose my mouth as its new primary target.

Another clinic meant another team of doctors, and even though they could read my history, they still didn't fully appreciate that I was 'one of those patients' that had already tried all the drugs, many times. They still wanted to start with the weak drugs and see if they worked. Even though it made sense as the disease was attacking a much smaller area, I knew deep down that these drugs wouldn't help. It was over four years until they eventually injected my lip with steroids (every two to three months) which finally returned it to a normal size; this involved pulling the lip down and injecting five or six times in a line just below the dry to wet transition area. My lip would swell up even bigger for about three days before slowly returning to a near-normal size for about eight weeks. Getting home after these injections became quite comical; in winter I would easily hide the triply bloated lip (the underlying inflammation, the swelling from the trauma of multiple neighbouring injections and the extra substance that had been added to the area via the injections) with a scarf, but in the hotter months I would cover it with a tissue - which would become bloody. I would get a lot of looks on the train, people thinking I had just been punched. On a couple of occasions, I was asked if I was ok, as I wasn't able to talk properly with the swelling and as the local anaesthetic hadn't completely wore off, I could only attempt a smile and nod.

I'm happy to say I do not require these injections anymore as my other inflammation treatments keep it at bay. I can still feel a hint of inflamed tissue below the surface of the lip, and on the very rare occasion it swells up for a few days, but on the whole it is contained and thankfully there is no lasting tissue damage.

Rewind to that summer, and it was time for me and my new lip to return to school; my cheeks were no longer swollen but the lip was very enlarged. I was very conscious of it; vanity played its part, but I also think that as I was so used to concealing and obsessing about something, it was my natural state of mind - particularly at school. It was bright red, more than four times the normal size and not symmetrical (much bigger on the left side); it clearly looked unnatural, even painful - botox gone very wrong. The lip on my mind added to the stress of starting with a new year group; I would cover it with my hand, look down to hide my face, or push it into my mouth in an attempt to hide it. It was still very obvious as the skin under the bottom lip stuck out like I was pushing my tongue there, and if I opened my mouth to talk it would fall or rather flop out.

I got more used to the bag at school, its timings (it usually fills up 30-60 minutes after eating) and generally having it in public. Once I had a bag that suited me (and therefore didn't need to change it at school), PE or more specifically the changing rooms were the only times I really had to worry about it. Even though I was becoming happier with it by this point, I didn't want to know what other people thought about it, so I would time taking my top off with when no one was looking, or if possible, face a corner. When clothed unless you are looking for it, you can't tell there is a bag there.

A meeting with my Head of Year also alleviated some other concerns. We talked through how the school could support me; with the workload (as I had been out of that world for a while) and with the new year-group integration, but from my perspective the best thing to come from the chat was that we arranged my access to the school nurse's bathroom - for me to empty and change my bag.

In hindsight this would have been helpful in my pre-surgery school years - access to an always clean and open toilet. But lesson learnt; other people can help…if you let them.

The first year back was okay, I kept to myself during lessons and could join up with my old year group at break times. After the initial period of questions about where I had been, which were still mostly answered with little detail and deflection, it was nice to get a taste of normality. It did feel a little like I was in limbo, knowing these renewed friendships would be short-lived.

The start of the second year back was much tougher, as my original year had now left the school. I was self-conscious with my lip as aggressive as ever, and still with little self-esteem. I remained withdrawn, not engaging much in lessons or with the other students. I spent quite a few break times back in the familiar toilets, but this time hiding. It was easier than standing around by myself in public view.

This didn't last more than a few months, over time I made some good friends - the people I sat next to in lessons, the boys on the bus, and my art class. They took me under their wing and we would even hang out outside of school. For the first time ever, aged eighteen, I started to do ordinary things with friends, my first real taste of independence - not the traditional 'from the parents', but from the toilet.

During that year, I slowly felt a transition away from worrying about the lip (and the bag), towards just being sick of being in a stressed-out state. It took long enough, but I was finally on the path to truly understanding it wasn't doing me any good and it really didn't matter.

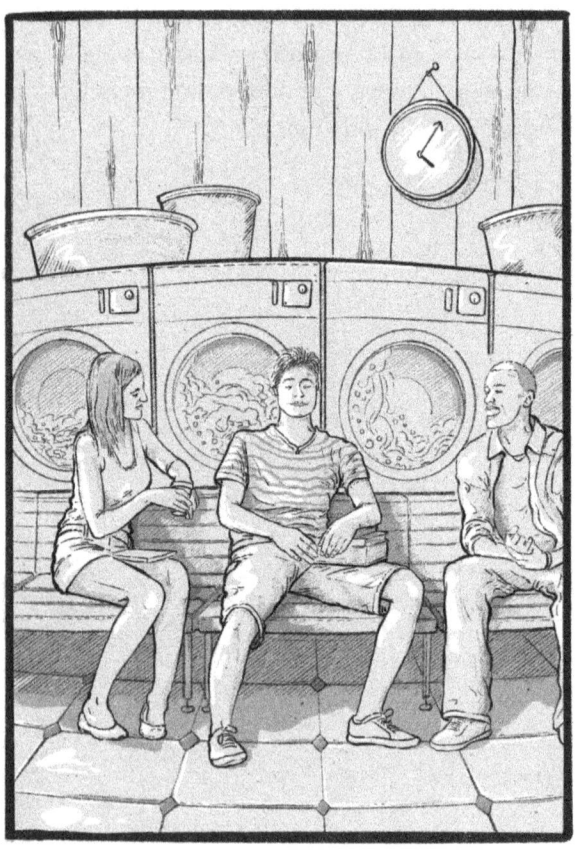

- A New Life! -

I did well enough in school to get into university and despite my mind's trained negative bias - pursuing things for me to overthink - I was looking forward to it. Even with the nuisance lip, I felt normal now, ready for a normal chapter in my life. The surgery had granted me the fresh start I had thought about; able to be myself more, feeling mostly free from the oppression of active Crohn's Disease.

Not that this book is about giving explicit advice, but one thing I fully endorse is that if your situation is similar to how mine was, you should not fear surgery. It took years to fully appreciate, but it transformed my whole life and I wish I had it sooner.

As my disease was now controlled and stable, there were much longer stretches of my life with less Crohn's related stories to share. Now it was less about struggling with the disease, and more about dealing with the inconveniences and little obstacles having a bag can bring.

After a long summer, moving out for university approached. I was allocated student accommodation in which I was sharing a single bathroom with a large number of people. Even though I had had the bag a couple of years now, this wasn't ideal; primarily I was nervous about the amount of time it took me to change the bag, thinking that for example in the morning when everyone wants to get in there and I'm taking that extra 10-15 minutes too long - I did not want that additional attention or pressure brought on my bathroom activities. I was also a bit concerned if the bathroom would remain clean enough.

Looking back, I'm sure I would have adjusted to the situation and it would have been fine, but it felt quite daunting at the time. After explaining my condition to the university, they were able to move me to a different building where the students had their own en-suite. It wasn't the luxury en-suite you may have in mind - at all - but knowing I would have my own small private space to create a new bag changing routine brought massive peace of mind. Other overthought topics included: What if people see my bag supplies? I kept them in a big chest, and I had this silly idea that people would question it and want to know the contents. How will I dispose of my bags without people seeing? Again, I had this illogical thought that people would notice that I would take out my bathroom bin more than average. And lastly, I worried that my slightly strange diet would be noticed and commented on.

I quickly made a group of friends, and had a full and proper social life - being normal was great! As before, I did not openly announce my disease (or bag) to my new friends, unless circumstance required it. One such situation arose two months in when my course took a trip to Barcelona. Similar to my concerns about halls, I wasn't in a place where I was comfortable sharing a bathroom with a hostel dorm of 16 relative strangers. After discussing with my tutor, to keep costs down and myself comfortable, a smaller room was deemed appropriate, for me and one other. Therefore, I had to tell a new friend on my course at a very early stage of our friendship.

We were at the bus stop alone when I chose to tell him. I kept it simple saying I had Crohn's Disease and a bag, and why it was difficult for me in the big dorm room. He had a few questions but it was very much like 'oh okay, no worries' and then we moved on - no big deal. It felt good not feeling like I had to hide it from someone, and as my confidence grew over the next months of university, I matured to the place that I wanted to tell people. Slightly contradictorily, I didn't like people knowing that I did not personally tell. It was different from my reservations at secondary school, it wasn't about toilet or pooing my pants embarrassment or even about judgement at all. I hated the idea of it being a piece of gossip. 'By the way, did you know Mike has a bag?' It may have been because I didn't want misinformation spread around - as the disease was still relatively 'new' to public knowledge at this time, but mainly because it was a traumatic experience that I felt shouldn't be just thrown into a conversation. I also loathed the idea of it being used to define me - by people that didn't know me; 'You know Mike?' 'I think so, the guy with a bag right?'

Now I don't care at all, I'll tell anyone anything... even write a book about it. I guess that's growing up - coming to terms with who you are - I just took a little longer to get there.

It almost became a badge of trust, once I had reached a level of friendship with someone, I would sit down with them and open up. It isn't a reflection on the people before, it required me getting to that level of self-confidence, as well as trusting the person. Before I trusted people, but wasn't ready myself. It was self-fulfilling, the more I confided in friends the more self-assured I became, reaching the point where I felt unembarrassed and fully relaxed about telling some of my more colourful stories.

It was best to have the conversation one on one in a private setting. I would keep the story short, in chronological order, highlighting what I thought was most relatable; starting with diagnoses at a young age, repeating the school year, and then to having my worst bits removed. If they were intrigued by any part, I'd answer their questions and elaborate, if they didn't understand what the surgery entailed, I'd explain that as my intestines can no longer connect to my rectum, they come out through my skin on my belly. The response was usually one of surprise, and it always ended with a big hug and stronger connection with the person.

Conflicting this, I often kept the illness out of friendships - for the first few years at least. This may have been a hangover from my adolescence where it acted as a barrier, but the real reason was because it was nice to have some friends 'away' from it. As the disease didn't dominate my life anymore, I didn't always think about telling a new friend or not - if it came up, it came up. This rings true today.

Besides making friends, living away from home, and not forgetting the studying, the other experience of university is of course partying and clubbing. Without my bag, I don't think I would have ever been able to enjoy even London's nightlife. Not enough toilets, too many people and alcohol would be too stressful. On the whole the bag didn't and doesn't affect anything about going out; I like to change it before leaving the house to be as fresh as possible, and may have to check once or twice that it is secure and not filling up too much throughout the evening. The only real hitch can be the security checks when entering a club.

Near my university there were multiple clubs but one very big one, which we would visit frequently. Usually the bouncers would just touch the outside of your pockets and then guide you through the scanner, which meant I didn't have to worry about drawing attention to myself in such a public setting. However, on one occasion a security guard gave a more thorough search and patted my front, feeling the bag. Instinctively I quickly moved my hand there to protect myself, and I assume with a startled and concerned look on my face said something like 'No!' or 'No, No, don't grab that!' The large bouncer grabbed harder on the site and firmly threw me down to the floor. In the middle of the entrance space I had bouncers on top of me while I was trying to explain it isn't a bag of drugs!

The stoma has no nerve endings so there isn't much feeling in the area, but it is a part of my body that no one else touches, so it is sensitive in the way that it is only used to being touched by myself. Therefore, it didn't physically hurt me (except for the big guys on top of me), it was more a feeling of shock, and distress that my stoma had been damaged.

They took me to a separate room; it took me about 20 minutes before I could look. My mind was racing: Will I need surgery again? What if the stoma has been pulled out or pushed in? And how was I going to explain this one to my friends - many of whom I hadn't told yet. Once I had calmed down, I had a look with the medical staff and everything was okay. In that particular club, after that incident, I built a relationship with the club's medic. I would ask the bouncer at the door to call for him, and I would be waved through. He would even escort me to the staff loos if I wanted.

Now, I make sure I have a quiet word in the doorman's ear before he does a body search. Sometimes I encounter a jobsworth, who will question me and want to see it. This is rare, only needing to flash the bag on a few occasions - especially in non-English speaking countries. Just the once have I had to fully lift my top up in front of the whole queue.

Having had the bag for a couple of years I was pretty confident in nearly all situations - when fully clothed anyway. In public, clothes hide you from all the questions and misjudgements. Sexual activities were one of the top categories I contemplated in the run up to the surgery. How was it going to affect my sex life?

Before the surgery I was scared about all the aspects - the mechanics (would it get in the way?), will body on body contact hurt it, will they want me to keep it well clear of them and whether anyone would even want to sleep with someone with a bag?

After, with a better idea of the what having a bag meant, the only fear left was the 'ew' reaction. Whether it was verbalised or not, I dreaded hearing that retort or seeing it in the face of a girl I liked. I understand that having a bit of insides on the outside can be hard for some people to fully grasp and is a bit 'icky', but nevertheless you pray you won't get an unwarranted overzealous reaction.

The first time with the bag was a big step in overcoming this. As it was someone I knew well and who knew all about my Crohn's well in advance, it took the edge off - a lot of stressing for no reason. In terms of the physical activity, the appliance caused no real issues at all, and hasn't since. No pain, no awkwardness, no getting in the way. The latter is another key facet I considered a lot in the lead up - what was I actually going to do with the bag during, as in how best to position it. There are many products designed to make things easier and plenty of advice online: special lingerie for ladies, pouch covers, taking Imodium to limit output, wearing the bag horizontally so it doesn't dangle close to the genital area, stoma caps which are basically tiny bags you put on the stoma before and change after, even stoma plugs that block the stoma preventing faeces from leaving the bowel.

Everyone will have their own preferences, but personally I think that many of the accessories out there are over the top. For me covering and support is enough for my partner and I to be comfortable. My process is making sure my day-to-day bag is empty and then simply folding it up into my abdomen waistband. This way the pouch is flat, comfortable, out of the way, and not requiring any real 'preparation'. I sometimes worry that when I pop to the loo (to make sure it is completely empty) I am risking 'ruining the mood', an extended pre-sex routine before every encounter, like having to change into a smaller bag doesn't seem convenient or merited; particularly when you apply this to a long-term relationship.

In the first years I would keep my t-shirt on as an extra security layer, not just for me, I used to worry that my partner was anxious about the bag. Whether it was them not wanting to touch it (even when fully covered), or if they were concerned about hurting me, either way I would rather their thoughts weren't on it. With one-off encounters, I sometimes didn't even mention the bag; saying that I recently had surgery so would prefer not taking my top off. In continuing relationships, as both parties became more comfortable together, the t-shirt wasn't needed anymore, with only the waistband remaining. Over time I realised that not presenting my bag as a gross thing that I am conscious of, encourages my partner to not have that perception either.

I would say 'body confidence issues' isn't a term that applies to me, I am happy with my body and don't fear personal judgement; the most embarrassing aspect of Crohn's and ostomy bags are people's misconceptions of them. The beach is another good example, I always wear a t-shirt on the beach (even though it is not really needed as there are many good ostomy swimwear options). I resent people passing ill-educated opinions, 'He has a bag, which has poo in it, I better keep a good distance away in the water.' In recent years there has been an increase in public exposure, online coverage and some clothing models with bags; this can only be good for the public's education - although it is only the first little steps in dampening the stigma. Greater awareness and understanding will help all of the ostomy community particularly in regards to body issues, and especially for the newcomers and younger members.

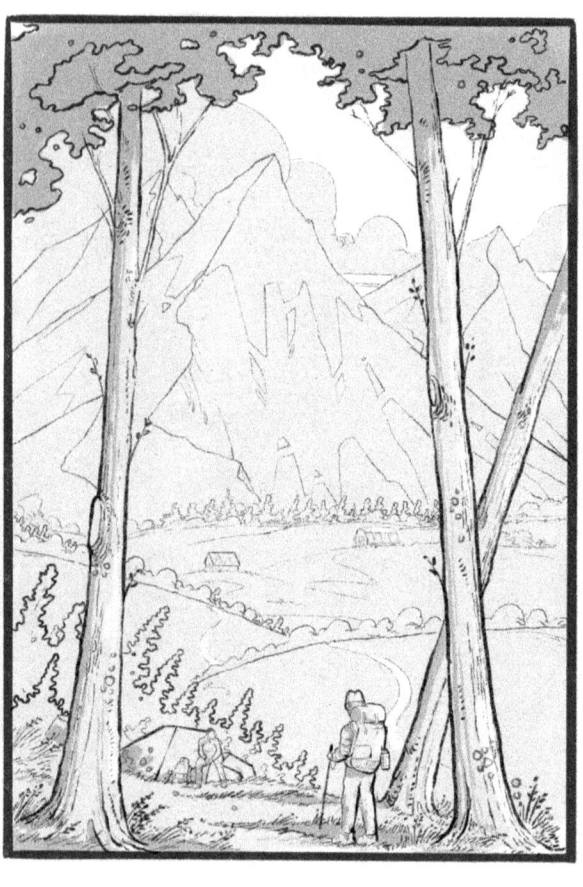

- All Crohn Up -

Moving into the world of work, I wasn't sure about the 'rules' of telling a possible employer about my disease. Am I supposed to tell them? How much detail? And at what stage - when applying or during the interview? I couldn't see it affecting my performance or the day to day, but did wonder if it was my duty to inform them that I was likely to have more days or half days off for hospital visits - for my lip treatment and other routine appointments and scopes. Was this going to affect my employability?

On my first contract there was a form which asked about medical conditions, I assumed for health and safety reasons. I answered with Crohn's Disease and OFG, there wasn't any follow-up questions or place to expand. I figured I am not the only one with a condition that MAY have a slight effect on their work, and I was fundamentally healthy now just with sporadic hospital commitments.

There were never any issues raised by the employer (when I had to take time off for hospital visits), at all, however from my side there was a sense of guilt when my appointments and treatments happened to cluster together - for example three to four days in a two-week period. Although not really my fault, I felt a little embarrassed that I was getting full pay but not putting in all the hours. For the shorter hospital trips - when I would be back in the office after about 3 hours, I would make-up the time by taking shorter lunches and staying later that week. But for the longer spells, primarily the lip injections (every 2-3 months) where it took some time for the lip to return to an acceptable level, so I could talk properly; it wasn't realistic that I could catch up two or three days of time out of the office. I would try to get appointments that would include the weekend in the (lip) deflating period, but it would still mean taking at least the Thursday and Friday off. After a few cycles, I became more sheepish and uncomfortable writing the email saying I will be off for a couple of days…again…for treatment.

I sought advice from friends and family, which mainly came back as 'don't worry about it', 'it is what it is', and 'I'm sure there are other people who take many more sick days than you.' Nevertheless, I was new to the work environment and I really liked my bosses and colleagues, so it continued to play on my mind. I proposed that when it wasn't just a quick appointment or a short half-day, that I would use some of my holiday days to offset the 'cost'. In the subsequent years I have realised this definitely was not necessary, there was no grievances or pressure from my employer, but for my very first experience of a professional employer-employee relationship it helped me feel more at ease.

I kept an 'in case of emergency' change of bag stored in my desk and there was a larger (disabled) toilet close by if I had to make a change. My colleagues didn't need to know details and my disease didn't affect anything; the office setting brought no Crohn's or bag related stress to a normal day. The only possibility of some embarrassment would be the farting noises my stoma would sporadically emit, but this was not constantly on my mind as I became better (I hope!) at controlling and minimizing this. I came to recognise the feeling of gas or poo getting close to the end of its journey. I would then place my hand on the bag (on top of my clothes), and position a finger over the opening of the stoma. When the content would be pushing out, the finger would prevent it erupting at a fast rate, slowing the flow normally dampens the sound. I've long forgotten the feeling, but apparently this is the same as clenching to control a bum fart. If the office is particularly quiet in that moment, or it felt like it could be a very loud one, I'd cough, or start a short conversation or maybe offer to make tea to mask it; if one slipped out unannounced... people usually just ignore it anyway.

Another unique and peculiar circumstance comes from the incontinence - having no control over when the stoma is active. It is strange enough sitting in the pub or at the dinner table casually chatting with friends or family, but I don't think too many people can say they have been in a meeting with their boss and an important client, while they are secretly having a poo under the table. The opposing experience is when I have a blockage. Once or twice a year I will wake up with very little output in the bag, and a bit of discomfort in my abdomen. Certain foods like popcorn can make this happen. For me a bit of stretching and walking around usually gets things flowing again; at its worse I would be a little late to work, having to walk around before going into the office.

There was one day when a water pipe had been hit by some local construction work, which cut the supply to a large area around the office. Suddenly no flushing toilets was a bit of a dilemma, there was still half the day left. With no capacity to 'hold it' and needing to use the facilities for number twos more than normal, I would have to empty my bag, and cover the contents with toilet roll. But the toilet was slowly becoming fuller and fuller with tissue paper; it overflowing when the water was back on would have been horrendous - and I thought I would have been the main contributor to this.

I should have explained to someone and gone home, but that would have been curious in a relatively small office. Without any other options, the toilets filled up and up until the end of the day, matched by my stress levels; the following morning they were empty so it all must have just flushed away without complications. Phew.

After a couple of years of working, now with a good few years of confidence building under my belt, a conversation with a colleague and friend who had just got back from travelling around India, caused me to reflect on my life so far. I had already missed out on quite a bit, and started to consider that my life choices, since my health had been put straight, weren't making the most out of it. An incredible urge instantly grew within to do something new and adventurous; I began to plan a lengthy trip away, thinking it would help me make up for some of the time I had lost to Crohn's.

It felt like India would be too much of a culture change - for my bowels at least. Westernised countries seemed like a more appropriate starting point; places where there would be more robust healthcare if something were to happen. I chose New Zealand and Australia. My doctors advised against it because of the risks, especially the extended period I was proposing - four months. I would be away from my doctors, and it would mean stopping one of the injections that I self-administered at home - as it needed to be constantly refrigerated, which after some investigation it became clear wasn't viable when backpacking - moving from place to place, hostel to hostel.

We discussed what it would mean to my treatment plan and how we could best negotiate a pause in the injections, I could easily continue with my other medications, which were just tablets at this point. Even though medically he couldn't advise it, the doctor understood that I couldn't (or didn't want to) let the bag or the disease stop me doing what I wanted to do.

I coordinated further with my IBD nurse, getting emergency numbers, action plans, and a note from the hospital in case my masses of tablets and provisions were questioned at customs. For extra peace of mind, I made sure my travel insurance covered the disease, and would, if necessary, fly me home in an emergency. I started to work out how many of each ostomy item I would need. All guidance was to take double the amount you would normally use in the time period. The reason for the excess is to cover yourself if you need to change the bag more regularly because of things like hotter weather (sweatier), if you do activities that might require extra changes, for example swimming every day, or if some go missing. It is also wise to split up the supplies when flying or when taking coach trips, with a few weeks kept with you as hand luggage - in case your main bag gets lost in transit.

Budgeting for one change of bag a day I laid out all the supplies I would need (under these guidelines) on the bed. It was clear there was no chance it would fit, even in my extra-large backpack - it was a massive heap of bags, adhesive rings, sprays and wipes. I re-packaged to condense what I could, and squeezed as much as possible into my large backpack; with every pocket completely wedged full - leaving only 30% for clothes - I managed to take approximately three months' worth. It was a nightmare zipping up the overflowing bag every time I opened it, but after a few weeks - as I used up the supplies - it obviously became easier to close and carry.

The plan was two months in New Zealand and two in Australia. The three month supply (according to the one change a day assumption) would have to last until I got to Melbourne, where my parents would ship - to a prearranged hostel - what I needed for the rest of the trip. If I was using too many bags in New Zealand (changing more than once a day), I would just have to be more conservative with them, and if the resupply was held up, at least I would be in a big 'modern' city where I was sure I would be able to find some supplies (even if not from my usual brand), and worst-case scenario I could fly home. My parents did have some issues getting the items through Australian customs - which they did not inform me about at the time, but after a lot of emails and calls the package went through.

This was a big step, it showed me how powerful the surgery was. Previously I could barely leave my house without crippling worries, and now I was heading to the other side of the world. It underlined that with some preparation, a bag can be managed and not restrict opportunities.

'Some' preparation may be an understatement here, the medical logistics was one aspect, but there was a lot of deliberation and anticipation alongside this. Thinking about new situations that I would likely come across, and devising the best way to deal with them. It's no surprise that bathrooms were the main factor I pondered.

At home I'm used to a typical bathroom; with a toilet, a sink and some surfaces on which I can place the various items I need for a bag change - a window sill, the sink surround, a shelf. I expected that most hostels would have shared toilet blocks - individual toilets in cubicles and separate sinks. For two reasons this kind of arrangement isn't ideal for a bag change. Firstly, there is no sink in the vicinity of the toilet, making cleaning the stoma site difficult (no clean water supply to wet the wipes). Secondly, the lack of surfaces in the cubicle - usually a plain, small rectangle with just the toilet and a small tissue paper dispenser.

My first solution was to just stay in dorms which have an en-suite (usually shared with 4 - 6 people), I figured these would be more 'normal' bathrooms, with a sink and toilet together; a private sink solves both problems, clearly providing water but also some space by the tap to put my changing kit. Alternatively, if this isn't possible, I could get a private room with my own bathroom.

To do this it looked like I would have to decide my route and book all my hostels in advance, as in the busier destinations these rooms were booked up weeks ahead. After some research and talking to some well-travelled friends, this strategy didn't seem feasible. It would have been far more expensive, require too much planning, and I was told that 'it just won't be like that, you will meet people and your route and timings in each place will change all the time!'

Back to the drawing board then, this time I tackled each hurdle separately. The water supply; a call to my ostomy supply company solved this in a matter of minutes. They make these mini spray bottles that can be refilled with water, as long as I changed the water every few days it would be clean. They also recommended some ostomy travel bags as a solution to the other problem, but these products were designed for storing equipment (a few changes worth) in an ordered way. Intended to prevent them being damaged rather than to assist the changing process.

I puzzled over this one for a while; an option could be to place the travel bag or some of the items onto of the tissue dispenser, but these could be too small, and it wouldn't be enough for all the items anyway. The floor wasn't hygienic, and stuffing some into my pockets wasn't really feasible.

With no ideas I started to look up if anyone had blogged about a similar problem, no luck here either. There were multiple reviews on travel kits for ostomy supplies but they were for more typical travelling - to other people's houses or to hotels - not for hostels and backpacking. I continued to browse and search, hoping to stumble upon anything useful. I came across a guy who was reviewing toiletry bags for hiking, and noticed that one of the bags had a hook (similar to the top of a clothes hanger). Eureka, I could hang the kit from the top of the cubicle wall! There may not be shelves but every cubicle would have a wall! The bag would easily fit 5 - 10 days' worth of supplies, it would stay hygienic and be easily accessible while hanging there.

I was satisfied with this solution - thinking I had all the angles covered - until about ten days before the flight out. Lying in bed I suddenly realised that it didn't work if the wall was very high or went all the way into the ceiling! Reassessing with the family we figured that taking something to hang it off would be best; a suction cup coat or towel hanger fit the bill. They are very cheap so I bought a few to test if they could hold the weight. I knew it was possible that I could encounter a toilet, which had walls to the ceiling, made from a material that the suction cups wouldn't stick firmly to, but I couldn't use this single circumstance as an excuse to cancel the trip - *even though I did briefly consider it.* This hypothetical cubicle was encountered in one hostel, I dealt with it by clumsily hooking the supply bag onto the neck line of my jumper, then awkwardly and slowly changed my ostomy bag. This predicament and investigation isn't particularly interesting, but it shows how something trivial for most people can be problematic to others. My preparations were so thorough and exhaustive because it was the first time; it was totally worth it and going travelling was one of the best decisions I ever made.

There were some things that I hadn't put much thought into that did require some adapting and getting used to. Sharing a room with ever changing people was the most notable one; over time I developed strategies to make myself more comfortable in that environment. First thing in the morning was the trickiest time, as this is the only time when my bag would be completely full and therefore clearly noticeable, even with clothing. So heading straight to the bathroom is always my first morning task. The simplest way to make this more discreet in a room full of people is getting a bottom bunk. This prevented me having to climb down a ladder (or jumping down) whilst trying to protect and hide a bulky, full bag sticking out of my abdomen. The other potential stumbling block is that most people in a hostel get up at similar times, usually timed with checking out or with the hostel's breakfast. To ensure I'd be able to get straight into a toilet (without queueing) I would set my alarm two minutes before the common wake-up time, for example 8:58 instead of 9:00. This way I was already out of the dorm room and in the toilet before the rest of the hostel woke up.

The bag impeded me with very few holiday or travelling activities, solely based around time between toilet facilities. Anything that would mean three or more hours without an opportunity to empty the bag wouldn't be doable; for example, some of the longer desolate hikes. I was able to climb mountains and go on expeditions lasting multiple days, but I would just have to make sure there was some sort of semi-private toilet facilities every few hours along the trail.

Fast forwarding a few years, I've discovered these 'travel disposable urinal packs', they are basically compact packets that contain an absorbing gel or powder. They are meant for you to urinate into, and the powder solidifies the liquid and neutralises any smells, and then it neatly seals and folds down. I can simply open my bag into the packet and be on my way. These have allowed me to go on full day climbs in remote landscapes, without any fears. The bag actually makes doing wild poos much easier and arguably more gracefully than my fully connected friends – no pulling trousers down, no awkward squatting and less mess.

The more physically intense activities, such as bungee jumping and sky diving, were a little worrying. I wasn't sure about the strain on the body, if this would affect the stoma or if the skin and muscles around it being stretched to an extreme would cause a problem, and if the harness would pose a risk to the stoma - sliding over it or pressing too hard on it. In these circumstances, talking and explaining the situation usually solved it. Whether it was just being reassured that it is fine (people with a bag had done it before) or working out an alternative, for example with the sky dive, they attached the harness and clips in a different configuration and we arranged a signal with the instructor so I could prepare my abdomen just before he pulled the parachute cord. Scuba diving was a little more complex as I wasn't sure how the pressure of being that far down was going to affect the bag, especially if there was some air in it but also just generally on the stoma. After some Googling, it was clear I needed to obtain a letter from my doctor 'signing it off' - not so straightforward from the other side of the world - but a few emails later and I was good to go, there were no problems at all.

Only on two occasions did things not go so swimmingly, both strangely on boats. The first was on the ferry crossing between New Zealand's North and South Islands. In the boarding waiting area looking down I noticed a small pea sized brown dot on my white t-shirt, after a quick surveying glance around, I lifted my top to have a quick check, my bag had a small leak, nothing major but it needed to be changed. I decided it best to wait to get on the ferry and not risk missing it, so I put a jumper on to hide the stain and waited. I knew it wasn't going to be the smoothest change (requiring extra cleaning as well as being on a moving vessel), so decided I was going to exercise my right to use the disabled toilet once aboard – the extra space and tap access make everything much easier. I went straight in, undressed and unpacked my bag kit and laid out what I needed. It was worse than I had suspected, although contained there was much more to wipe away than normal, this was going to take at the very least 15 minutes, and I also needed to soap and rinse the small stain on my top. About three minutes in I was topless and peeling the bag off, when there was a knock at the door. I could see from the shadow underneath the door that there was a wheelchair user waiting. Shit.

I couldn't really explain the situation through the door, and wouldn't be able to on my way out (I wasn't going to flash them my bag!), they would see a 'fully abled' person leave and would judge me as a horrible human being. I was panicked, rushing to get clean and get a new bag on. They kept knocking, each time sounding more annoyed. Did they see me go in and are ready to have a go at me? Surely there is another disabled loo? I kept thinking I was putting this person in what used to be my worst nightmare - being unable to get to the toilet. I skipped some steps and clumsily threw a new bag on - it would hopefully see me through to my next accommodation. I opened the door, and timidly apologised before jumping out of their way… and then vacated the area as quickly as possible.

A moral / ethical debate this one. Should I have felt guilty? Did I need to apologise? Should I have changed in the conventional toilet? Even though ostomates (awful name!) do qualify as one of the invisible ailments that are permitted (assuming New Zealand has similar rules to the UK).

I don't have the answer, it was just unlucky timing really. The label "hidden" is used for illnesses in which individuals often suffer in silence, or show no immediately apparent signs, generally leading to misunderstandings among the general public. However, being hidden can have some benefits, not being visually diagnosed and pigeonholed by strangers being the main one, but this was definitely a rare situation I wished mine was more evident.

The other boat was a much smaller catamaran type, on a three-day sail around the Whitsunday Islands off Australia's East coast with around 15 other backpackers. On the second day we had a long snorkelling session chasing turtles and gawping at reefs, when back on the boat I suddenly felt a bit off and absolutely shattered, so went for a lay down in the hull. Upon waking up, I felt even worse and my mouth felt strange… my lip had exploded again - the lengthy exposure to salt water had triggered it (after this I realised I'm allergic to sea salt). I was stranded many miles away from my doctor, my emergency medicines and any phone signal. I only brought my standard tablets as we were supposed to pack light and I hadn't thought something like this was going to happen!

Covering my lip, I gingerly sauntered up on deck to the captain and asked if there was a satellite phone (hoping to consult my hospital). There wasn't, and with his shock at the size of the swelling, he asked if we needed to head back now… even though it would still take at least half a day to get there. I of course did not want this. Once the initial surprise had worn off and I had thought through my plan of action once back on land (getting the okay from my nurse or doctor before taking my safety-net steroids), I was able to get on with enjoying the tour. It wasn't my most comfortable expedition, but it was what it was. I had only met everyone on board the day before and they were great, obviously intrigued but also offering their help. A week later the lip had returned to normal and this was just a small blip on an amazing four-month experience.

As big as booking and setting off on this first adventure was for me, the experiences gained perhaps helped me even more. By the end my confidence with my disease, with my bag and in myself skyrocketed. I was able to be completely open about all of it to anyone, even if only knowing them a day or two. I had proved to myself that the disease truly did not have a hold on me anymore; still a part of me but just a meagre passenger.

As soon as I got home, fuelled by my new levels of self-esteem, I looked into my next trip; I saved for six months and was off, this time to Canada for three months. Here I met my girlfriend, the writer of the 'Dating Crohn's' chapter. After this trip it's safe to say I had caught the 'travel bug'. I deferred my Masters course and saved up again.

This time South America was the destination. Asia, more specifically South-East Asia was the first choice, but the hygiene and gastro diseases in that area were too risky. South America was a compromise, middle ground; the doctors still advised against it, but knew I was going to go.

Being less 'westernised' brought new hurdles, (access to healthcare / hygiene standards / the water / vaccines) but that just meant extra planning and extra precautions. I got all the vaccines I needed and as many of the additional ones I was able to have - with a compromised immune system there are some vaccines, 'live' ones, that I am unable to have - for example against yellow fever. A weakened immune system just meant I had to be clever with my route, namely avoiding high-risk malaria zones - which most people do anyway.

I got my doctor's notes translated into Spanish, researched the best ways of treating drinking water, and looked into the smart choices for buying and preparing food. There was also the issue that whatever water was not safe to drink, I shouldn't be cleaning my stoma with it either; a bit more research and found out that most travellers only drink bottled water. So, I just made sure I always kept a spare small bottle close by, or at least knew where a close by shop was. Preparation was now second nature, not needing to predict and scrutinize all potential situations anymore.

I was more lenient with my guidelines on this trip, not letting my three-hour rule prevent me from doing any activities or staying with the group of friends I had made. I started to 'wing-it' trusting myself to adapt (or just deal with the consequences) if I had to. Instances that come to mind are risking the Death Valley cycle ride without knowledge of any facilities on the isolated route, or heading into a giant silver mine not knowing for how long, and definitely knowing there are no toilets down there. Finally, and pertinently, one that I was setting myself up to fail was the toilet-less night buses; leading to me having to empty my bag in darkness by the side of the road, surrounded by elderly Bolivian ladies squatting themselves. Dignity is overrated.

Sorry for banging on about travelling, but it was a huge part of getting to where I am with my disease. It enabled me to confront my deep-lying fears and beat them by being far outside my long-lived comfort zone.

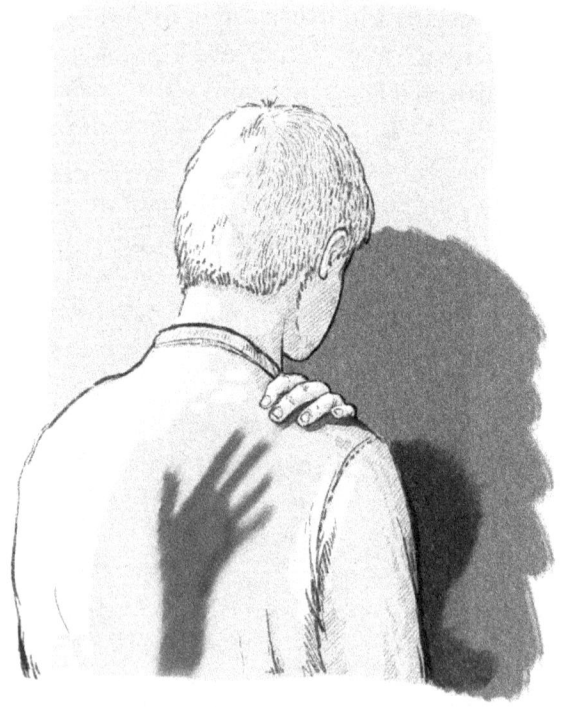

- Mental Flares -

Back in London I returned to 'normality', working and finally taking my place on my Masters course (and of course still always planning my next adventure in the background). On the whole, life was pretty good, especially as the girl I met in Canada finally moved to London to live together!

She has been my sounding-board whilst writing this book, helping me select which experiences to share and pushing me to dig down into the feelings behind them. These conversations and when discussing her chapter, highlighted to me a way the disease may still be playing a part in my life that I hadn't previously put much thought to - my depressive tendencies. To this day I have episodic waves of 'very low mood', I'm wary of using the word depression as I've never formally been diagnosed - but my symptoms very much align with it. I'm fully aware I should have and should speak to a professional about it! But I guess I just don't want to spend any more time with doctors and appointments. But still, stupid man and dumb excuse.

Things like travelling and university were great distractions from it, so I never really noticed the pattern or thought of myself in that light. But after being settled in a more typical life routine the semi-regular sequence of dropping into a depressive state every few months became noticeable - especially to my girlfriend.

I would become incredibly fed up with life, not wanting to do anything, or talk to anyone, barely eat and just be surrounded by tiredness and negative thoughts - sometimes completely unable to get out of bed.

I'd lay there thinking 'why now?', 'how am I here again?', 'why can't I snap out of this?' and that 'I'm wasting more of my life stuck in a room again'... sending me into a spiral. This deeper state usually lasted just a day or two, but the general slow dive into it and re-emergence usually being around five to ten days.

Eventually I started to talk to others about it - mainly my girlfriend but also to two friends with diagnosed depression and who have really struggled with it in the past. Although not linked to chronic illness, there is a lot of crossovers with our thoughts and we discuss the triggers and generally just try to talk it out with each other. Just talking about how crap the thoughts and feelings are instantly helps. We have a mini-pact to message in the group chat if things are getting bad and we usually check in every now and then.

This is the polar opposite to those tough teenage years, I bottled everything up and struggled alone with a lot of the mental battles. Perhaps an outlet like this would have been a great help - maybe a doctor, a therapist, a teacher or a friend. But at that age I couldn't see, I kept these hidden torments secret as much as I could - mine to hate and mine to deal with. I don't recall being offered this sort of help from the hospital or from the school (whether I would have accepted it or not!) but I hope this is now part of the care for young people with Crohn's and other chronic illnesses.

Chronic illness is known to be linked with depression, but I've never thought my Crohn's had much to do with mine - not directly anyway, not anymore. Again, never diagnosed, but my teenage isolation and state of mind was definitively depressive and linked or even caused by the situation the disease put me (and my family) in. But it's not something I actively think about in my healthy years, so personally don't hold it to account for this… although I do concede it may have played a part in creating a stronger negative bias in my brain.

One of the key reasons depression and chronic illnesses are associated is the life-long aspect - it staying with you for the rest of your time. So sticking with Crohn's, I assume people who get the disease later in life have life-experience and pre-disease memories of a time that they 'miss', and may not be able to fully get back to. This frustration or mourning gets them down, plays on their minds or they are overwhelmed by this fact - feeling hopeless or helpless. For me it's almost the opposite, I don't have a time I miss healthwise, I'm living the good period!

In the recent years the only other real reminder of my Crohn's was the Covid-19 pandemic. I don't want to dwell on it (as we have all heard enough about the Coronavirus!) but I wanted to touch on my experience as an at-risk person.

Being an autoimmune disease, with common treatments being aimed at suppressing the immune system, the virus had a big impact on my life and the IBD community. With two of my long-term medications being immunosuppressants, I fell in to the extremely vulnerable risk group and had to 'shield'. This basically meant no or absolutely minimum contact with anyone outside the household – directly or indirectly. i.e. if a household member left the house for work you had to completely isolate from them *and* everyone in the household they interacted with.

As our flat was too small to be able to follow shielding advice for 'in-household' social distancing, my girlfriend also had to shield to protect me. Sticking to the guidance and with no garden we were inside the flat for nearly 3 months - with my parents dropping off food at the doorstep every other week. Then followed a further six months of the same but with one walk to the park every day.

I'm trying my best to not use this small section to fully vent about the frustrations and anger ...but very quickly... looking out the window or hearing about friends (and politicians) blatantly breaking the rules was incredibly difficult, especially whilst we (and many others) were trapped inside with no plan and no end in sight for us.

Being locked in took me back to the isolation of my teenage years almost being comfortable in an extended period of loneliness and depression.

At the time of writing, my 'down' periods have massively decreased again and are a very small part of my life. I've learnt to recognise the signs of the negative thoughts creeping in and have tried to fill my time with things that keep me busy and make me happy. Returning to sport being a massive one, running around a football pitch making jokes with friends is the ultimate happy place for me... it's true what they say about exercise and socialising being a great remedy!

- No More Secrets -

Nearly 25 years ago our mission was to control Crohn's until I made it to adulthood…we failed in that but got through it and came out the other side strong. I look back at old photos in shock, 'did I really look that ill!', I have come a long way from hiding the bloody toilet bowl from my parents.

I've now had a bag for over 15 years! And will happily have it for another 50. A common question I get asked is 'How long will you have the bag for – when will it be reversed?' but after the first year, there was never a thought to 'going back', why would I risk what it has given me. Looking down at it now, I wonder where I would be without it. Unquestionably it has changed the course of my life, opening up so many doors which used to be firmly locked.

It is impossible to overlook the profound impact Crohn's has had on me, diagnosed so young the challenges that followed have made me resilient, played a big part in shaping my character, provided me with life perspective, given me a strong understanding that you can't control everything and perhaps most importantly showed me (eventually) that being open is the best policy.

The unpredictability and spread of Crohn's (as well as the additional risks it brings with other more scary things!) make the future cloudy, but I'm very optimistic that the worst is definitely behind me, and if it isn't I am more than prepared to face it. If a heavy relapse destabilises me or another operation is required, whether to remove my rectal stump or something more serious, I do not fear it. I take steps by trying to live healthy to avoid or delay the potential hurdles, but I've accepted whatever may come.

I hope this book helps in a small way to break down some of the stigmas. It is encouraging to see that hidden diseases are now starting to get more attention and some understanding. With these sorts of things, public misconceptions are key in repressing open conversations – publicly and with those close to sufferers.

Awareness of Crohn's has most certainly increased over the last two decades, with responses going from 'oh what's that?' to 'oh yes I've heard of that', but bags are lagging behind especially in terms of what they actually are. The 'fear of misjudgement' is an absolutely enormous weight on the people having to go through it, especially for younger people in the run up to the surgery. So hopefully my experience has shined some reassuring light on this!

Sharing my story has been empowering and a real therapy for me. I've been reminded of things long forgotten or subconsciously buried deep down, my eyes have also been opened to the extent and magnitude of the burden those dark years put on those around me.

I hope my story has also helped you in some small way - whether you are a patient, a doctor, a friend or relative. Or at very least I hope it has provided some tips and improved your knowledge. To those currently in the trenches battling a chronic illness, know you are not alone and please learn from my mistakes, seek support! Don't suffer alone.

No More Secrets

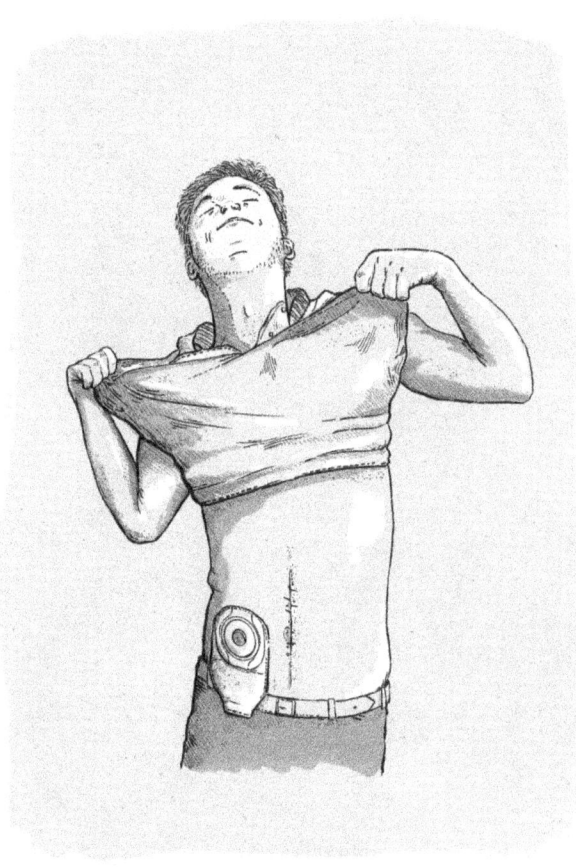

Appendix

Appendix

- Parental Guidance -

I understand families will do anything for you and can appreciate and see my family's support over the years. Whether it's my mum clearing up my projectile vomit at 3am and metaphorically holding my hand through everything; my step-dad taking me to school when I couldn't get on the bus, and always encouraging me to get out of my room; my grandad driving me to hospital when I couldn't face the underground; or my grandma keeping me company on my hour-long toilet visits when I was little. Nevertheless, not being a parent myself I have no real concept of what having an ill child is like.

In the worse years, being so young and consumed by the disease, I couldn't comprehend the affect it had on those closest to me. Over the course of writing this book, I questioned my parents, probing for things to jog my memory. They found it quite difficult reliving some of the ordeal but it quickly became clear to me that their experience - much of which was news to me - should also be shared!

From the extensive notes my mum wrote out, we condensed it into the following questions and answers.

What were the most difficult times?

The undiagnosed initial period was difficult; seeing my child suffer and not knowing what was wrong. We were terrified of the test results, our world had been turned upside down. My beautiful son had been diagnosed with a life-long chronic illness. To see your child suffer in pain is indescribable. I was devasted, shocked and heartbroken.

There was fear and sadness as I came to terms with his illness. As a mum I wanted to protect him and keep him safe; I knew I had to find a way to manage my own pain and emotions, stay physically and mentally strong, for the wellbeing of Michael, and to help him manage this debilitating disease. I wished I could take his pain and put it in me.

I asked myself many questions: Should I get another opinion? Can I do more? Did I do something wrong? Are there alternative treatments or medicines? Will he always have to struggle? For how long? Can it get worse? How is Michael really feeling? Will I live in constant fear?

His struggles deeply saddened me, but I couldn't fix it or take the pain away, we had to accept it and try to make life better for him; taking it one day at a time otherwise it became too overwhelming.

Are there any really specific memories?

The relapses were the most memorable times, when the disease was very active. His immune system attacking his own body, stomach pain, vomiting, diarrhoea, no appetite, weight loss, fatigue, very pale, very weak, very quiet and withdrawn. Not knowing day to day how he was feeling inside was tough. We supported him fully, reassuring him as much as possible that the flare-ups are temporary.

We tried to not project fear and anxiety. Swallowing tears and staying strong for Michael - this was draining and exhausting at times. It was extremely upsetting to see him suffering; unable to go to school, or do daily tasks, spending many hours in his room with no energy. We tried to focus on what he could do rather than what he couldn't.

What was the impact on the whole family and family life?

It was a balancing act, looking after Michael and helping him manage however we could, whilst ensuring we spent quality time with his brothers. I didn't want them to feel neglected. I explained to them that I would have to devote more time to Michael because of his illness, but they were just as important and loved the same. We talked about his condition and surgery, and shared our worries and concerns; it was ok not to be ok. It was important they knew what was happening to their brother. The disease was not going away, and he needed our help.

We learnt to ride the emotional rollercoaster, good days and bad days. The family would adapt to how he was feeling; low energy / low moods, we'd try to be calm and patient with him, and try to understand why. But, it is inevitable that emotions will swing; powerlessness, anger, frustration, guilt, anxiety.

It was important to make the most of the periods when he was in remission; visiting family, friends and encouraging sports. When he wasn't in remission, we had to cancel or postpone many days out and family holidays until he felt better, we had to change to an earlier flight home on one occasion as he was very ill. Managing and negotiating his disease together as a family was key. Even with the unpredictability of the disease we were determined that Crohn's was not going to hold him or his family back. Our big family holiday to Florida was a good example - pre-surgery. Michael wasn't in deep relapse but wasn't in proper remission either. He wanted us to go, it was a trip all the boys had been looking forward to for a long time - the theme and water parks! We managed together, we went around the parks together, acknowledging where the closest toilets were and adjusting when he knew he just had to be near one for a while. Many times, mid-queue, he would have to go to the loo; one of us would just wait with him until the rest had finished on the ride. There was one day he didn't feel like he could go to the park, no problem, I stayed with him while my partner and his brothers went, and we reunited later.

There was a lot more to deal with in a normal week or month - days spent at home when Michael was unable to go to school, collecting him from school when he became suddenly unwell, taking him to school by car when he just couldn't get on the school bus, all the hospital appointments, stays and treatments. I was having to leave work early, take personal calls and leave in the middle of the day and take whole days off. To be able to deal with all the unexpected events and relieve the pressure and stress, I took a career break.

It was a huge weight off my mind. I could focus all my energy and time to looking after Michael and the rest of the family, I could be ready when they needed me. My family needed security and stability; keeping family life as normal as possible.

Let's talk food?

His lack of interest in food was frustrating and worrying. When the disease was active, eating made his symptoms worse, so he had absolutely no interest in food. Michael was very thin and it was difficult to reach his ideal weight. We had a constant concern about his diet; wanting to make sure that he was getting all the vitamins and minerals he needed to stay healthy and grow, but the foods triggering his symptoms made it hard. We would try to keep a record of the food he ate if he was unwell after eating.

We learnt to keep calm at meal times, relaxing rules and letting him eat what he 'fancied' when he was ill - so that he was eating something! And would encourage healthier foods when he was in remission.

How and where did you seek advice and information?
What support did you receive?
Did you confide in other parents or friends?

At the time of the diagnosis Crohn's and Colitis wasn't as well documented, especially in children. With all the hospital visits I formed a good relationship with his paediatric consultant and the nurses on the ward. I asked many questions, recording all the answers on paper, keeping detailed records of all medicines and tests - doses and dates. Questioning, learning and researching the condition helped us cope and feel more in control, less anxious and less depressed.

Having a supportive relationship with the medical teams helped Michael and the family come to terms with the disease and keep life as normal as possible.

Reaching out to other parents who had and continue to go through a similar experience was a great help and relief. I spoke in hospital and on the phone to other parents about how we can help our children, and how we were coping with a chronically ill child; sharing our emotions and concerns, experience and knowledge on treatments. Accepting the reality of having a child with a chronic illness puts other life issues into perspective. In the later years, when we were on the ward, his nurses would ask if we would speak to other children, and their parents, about coping with the disease. We had been through almost all of the treatments and had so much experience with the emotional turmoil of the disease. They believed we could provide hope to other families.

My partner, parents and friends were invaluable after Michael's diagnosis and through all the hard years. Helping with school runs for his brothers, taking us to hospital appointments, and all the emotions. I spent hours talking and crying about seeing my boy suffer. A support network of family and friends was so important in keeping fears and anxiety and pain in control.

Being a member of Crohn's & Colitis UK was valuable, using the information provided and reading about other people's experiences was extremely helpful. It gave us confidence in dealing with the disease and the surgery, it let us know we were not alone; real stories, real people, real fears. Worries shared!

Advice summary for parents:

- Build a relationship with the consultant and nurses.

- Keep detailed records: treatments, medicines, symptoms, response and remission times.

- Research and keep up to date with treatments.

- Emotional & mental support: join support groups, speak to other parents, share experiences, use your friends and family support network.

- Try to get your child to communicate how they are feeling, physically and mentally.

- Try to build your child's confidence: hobbies, holidays, family gatherings, friends.

- Speak to their school about their needs.

- Do not fear the operations - and try to install that into your child.

- Encourage a healthy diet and exercise - and try to track if any foods cause a flare-up, pain or sickness.

The surgery was a key episode, what was that experience like?

Over the years, Michael never complained and took it all in his stride, but I knew there was a better life for him.

That January was the tipping point, all the treatments that put him into remission no longer worked. He had no energy, was unable to go to school, constantly in pain and being sick, he was getting weaker and weaker. It was hard to bear, so upsetting to see him suffering. I talked, discussed, cried to my partner, my parents and friends about Michael's quality of life. I trusted and accepted the medical teams' words - that surgery was the best option to improve it.

I knew of his deep fear of the bag, so had to stay strong and positive when the words 'he needs surgery' were said to us. I did my best to reassure him that it will be ok.

I had concern for Michael's mental health. I wanted him to see, before and after the procedure, that it would relieve him of pain, let him eat, grow and live, instead of merely surviving. It would be a life-changer.

I was anxious and afraid of how he would cope with a bag; but seeing how he had managed his disease, I knew he would find the strength and courage to come to terms with the bag and the stoma. Especially when he would start to live his life again, the one Crohn's had taken away from him.

Knowing the upside of the procedure didn't make it less scary, they were going to cut him open after all. Talking through concerns with the surgeon and his amazing nurse Laura, lowered the psychological stresses. I spoke separately with Laura: how is Michael really feeling, he isn't talking much, is the surgery right for him? It was a very challenging period; I couldn't eat or sleep. Seeing him so ill while worrying about the surgery, and not projecting this onto him.

The morning of the operation I found an inner strength, I was determined, adamant I'd stay strong and positive, and make it clear to Michael that this surgery will finally make him fitter and healthier. The fear was written all over his face and my heart was beating. Holding back the tears, I focused on positive thoughts - putting on a coping façade for the doctors and Michael. Laura could sense my pain. 'It is ok to cry and be sad' she whispered to me.

I felt physically sick whilst he was in the theatre, watching the clock all the time. It was a huge relief when it was over, seeing him in the recovery room. The days leading up had been extremely agonizing and testing for everyone. The surgeon explained it was Crohn's not Ulcerative Colitis (there had been some uncertainty before); he explained Michael's disease was severe, the removed large colon was very inflamed and scarred - he will feel so much better very soon. All my emotions came flooding out.

Our concerns were now solely on how Michael would deal with the bag. Would he accept it? How will he react when he wakes up? I knew it wouldn't be easy to accept such a change, he would mourn the way his body used to be. The days after the surgery he was very weak and withdrawn; he couldn't even look at his bag or stoma. Getting through those first few weeks and months was tough. His confidence and self-esteem were very low. My son is a fighter, he had already battled with this disease for many years, he is resilient, driven and determined. Staying positive and with the support and encouragement of his outstanding team of surgeons, doctors and nurses, and by taking one step at a time, setting small targets, he would adjust to living with a stoma. We would get through this.

In hospital his stoma nurse was impressed by the speed with which he learnt to clean and change his bag. The more knowledge he gained about caring for his ostomy, his confidence slowly grew in accepting and managing it. My pain was gradually lightening too; I was so proud, it had been the right decision, he would cope!

Before leaving the hospital, we spoke to a psychologist about managing the emotional side of the surgery and living with a bag - stress, anxiety and depression. Michael was nervous about coming home, he grew to feel safe in hospital with the team supporting him. It was my job now to make him feel safe and protect him. An open and honest environment at home would help him adjust and get life back to some normality. When and whoever Michael decided to tell about his operation and show his stoma to, was his decision. Him being comfortable enough to open up was a massive step for everyone.

Speak on the longevity of the disease, how was handling it without any real remission for nearly 8 years?

The treatments became routine for Michael, he has shown amazing courage in dealing with the procedures: blood and stool samples, the scopes, enemas, MRI's, Barium Meals, Ultrasounds, CT scans, the laxatives and bowel preps. We were there to support him with all the uncomfortable tests, unpleasant medicines and embarrassing tubes. I put all my energy into getting him better. His pain is my pain.

He found the right balance between putting on a brave front and being true to his emotions – a coping tool for the journey of his chronic illness. He attacks every knockback - the diagnosis, the treatments, the tests, the fear of foods, surgery, oral Crohn's and his forced isolation from Covid-19 - with bravery and strength. He doesn't moan and just moves on to the next chapter.

Crohn's is life long, so I worry about Michael every day. I wear a protective shield and simply pray and hope that he will have a happy, healthy life, and continue to fight his battles in a positive way. He deserves a good life.

It is clear that he is winning his battle with the disease. His family will always be there to help and support him if it throws something new at him. He has shown us all what is important in life; health, family, love, happiness and strength. 'Our hero'- how his grandad describes him.

After reading about Michael's experience from his perspective, is there anything that surprised you? Would you change anything you did? Would you approach anything differently?

The overwhelming feeling is sadness, sadness that he was going through so many things that we were unaware of, and sadness that he was unable to tell us about many of the physical and mental pains.

I wish he'd been offered more support from specialists for the mental health side. If more information had been given to us, or the schools maybe we would have been in a better place to help him cope.

The most obvious change we would have made would be to try harder to convince Michael that surgery wasn't the hideous catastrophic outcome he feared. He suffered for far too long and the whole family agrees that having the operation earlier would have saved a lot of suffering.

The other overpowering feeling we got from reading the book was pride. We are so proud of how he dealt with the disease and hope his journey can help many others.

Appendix

- Dating Crohn's -

Mike and I met while travelling in beautiful western Canada. I had just finished university and was travelling with a friend for the first time. Despite what he might say, Mike definitely made the first move. His confidence, good humour and carefree personality charmed me and even after only a short time together, we decided to give a long-distance relationship a shot. His love of life and his desire to experience it to the fullest were contagious and just what I needed.

From the very first instance, there was nothing about Mike that could have revealed the illness he lives with or the burden from his past experiences with Crohn's. He exuded a joy of living that one rarely sees. With time and many conversations, I slowly started grasping the extent of everything he had been through – really putting into perspective how much I took my close to perfect childhood for granted. Even to this day, while helping with this book, I am surprised at some of the many stories I hadn't yet heard, really highlighting how much and for how long this disease had affected all aspects of his life.

It's crazy to think that I spent my teen years worrying about fitting in and what people thought of me while Mike dealt with the same things but magnified by the fear of people misconstruing his disease. Not to mention the physical pain, the isolation and loneliness that 16-year old me could never understand. It is clear that he's decided to not dwell too much on the past or the years that this invisible disease have taken from him and instead enjoy the better life his ileostomy bag has opened up for him. He has no real hate or resentment; he got some lessons on life that most of us only understand later or never do. Yes, he hasn't let his illness define him, but it has undeniably played a role in shaping him and his unique character. He turned it completely around; what once restricted him has now given him the courage to get out of his comfort zone. He doesn't waste any time on things he has no interest in.

Having done my degree in Immunology, I was probably more aware of Crohn's disease than most people and thought I understood Mike's experiences when he first announced it to me. But there is such a jump from knowing about a disease and knowing how to live with a life-long disease. I am a bit of a worrier, particularly when it comes to health, so early on I did spend some time online researching the impacts of the illness on long-term health (such as links to colon cancer – which at the time I thought was the only reason for someone to have a bag), and the common medications and their effects, because I worried what it all meant for Mike's health. This Google search, even though intended to reassure me about the condition, was fruitless and I soon realised that I couldn't let this define our relationship either. I thought about asking these questions to Mike (about the future implication of his disease) but never did as it became clear that I didn't need to know the answers as no one can predict what's to come anyway. I was also pretty sure Mike had made the conscious decision to not dwell too much on things he has no control over.

I ask questions about medications, about appointments, enquire if they are frequent enough, and help prepare questions for his doctors. He doesn't get annoyed at my questions and my involvement - it is my way of being supportive.

The only somewhat visible sign of his illness is the bag. It really didn't and doesn't bother me. I didn't know anyone with one and had no real preconception. Knowing that it had helped Mike to massively reduce his symptoms, made this clever solution seem like a great compromise. He showed me the bag early on and soon enough I was curious to see the actual stoma which again I found very impressive. The bag really is a remarkable piece of kit; on our first beach holiday together, Mike let the big waves throw him around and smash him into the shore without any thought of protecting it. I was so scared the waves would rip the bag open or off, or damage the stoma, but it stayed on with no leaks and no issues. Despite carrying the bag at stomach level, it isn't something he or I think about a lot, he is very confident in himself and in his body - at least at this stage in his Crohn's crusade. I wasn't there when he was going through the experiences he writes about, or the ones that are 'a bit much' to make this book, but I can see the results of the journey. He refuses to let the bag get in the way of a good time.

I think the openness around something quite personal helped us to get comfortable around each other very quickly. We can talk about bowel movements at any time of the day and it's never awkward. In fact, no one can bring up humiliating poo stories to a group of strangers, in the middle of a full pub, with so little embarrassment as Mike can. And even though some aspects of the disease will always have an impact on his daily activities, I would say I am mainly a supportive bystander to the Crohn's part of Mike's life. There will always be things that make our relationship slightly more quirky than other couples, like me keeping him company when his 'phantom poo' urges call him to the loo, or the laughs we have at the weird fart noises his bag randomly produces - which usually have great comedic timing.

One of the things I've had to learn was when and how or even if to mention or bring up Mike's Crohn's disease to others. I didn't initially know how to handle this, should I tell my friends when I talk about Mike? Or is this something personal that I have no business in sharing with others? I knew it didn't define him so why bring it up? It was always clear that it was not my place to talk about his experience to people he might not want knowing. But it has still shaped so much of his character so why hide it? And the disease no longer has a strong hold on his life so why keep this part of him a secret? I came to realise that my boyfriend's 'out of the ordinary' toilet habits aren't really anyone else's business.

I have found that there are contrasting reactions between knowing someone's got Crohn's disease and knowing they have an ileostomy bag. Talking about Crohn's feels less invasive as people don't usually know much about it and won't push further when told it's an inflammatory life-long illness as they quickly realise it's more than they bargained for. But talking about the bag – which I have only done with others very few times – people immediately bring their own assumptions, and it leads to more personal questions about bowel movements, hygiene and (mis)conclusions are often drawn. It's easy to not bring up the bag as it is very hard to notice anyway.

I've learnt that he isn't opposed to me telling people that he has Crohn's, but is uncomfortable with people knowing about his food traumas. I think it's because he has fully come to terms with the Crohn's, but he is still somewhat working through the food issues. He sees the phobia as irrational or thinks others will see it that way, or at the very least it would require a long explanation to make it relatable. This is probably one of the few times that I get annoyed at him. What's most frustrating is that after going through everything he did, it seems silly to me to let food hold him back. I still struggle with finding balance in how honest and open to be about his peculiar eating preferences when invited over for dinner or to a restaurant, particularly if they haven't met Mike. Before committing I need to find out what type of food will be served or look up the restaurant's menu and unless it is a safe option like a pub, I will always check with or for Mike first. It is a question of leaving worries behind and actually enjoying the outing, it is unfair to put him in situations where he isn't able to have some control. Which I completely understand. Although Mike may have a slightly more precarious relationship with food than other IBD sufferers, I assume this situation isn't unique.

To Mike's dismay (not really), I am a massive foodie and have spent many hours questioning him about his alien views on food and his unadventurous taste buds. It clearly goes beyond fussy eating and it is easy to see that it's strongly rooted in unpleasant past experiences. He remains the only person I've met that didn't even know what eggs tasted like. Don't worry he does now... and loves them.

On one of Mike's first trips to Montreal, we went to a nice restaurant and he ordered some grilled chicken, switched the rice for some chips (as he refused to eat rice – thankfully now another thing of the past) and quietly accepted the grilled veggies that came with it, to not look too demanding to the waiter. The plate arrived, the chicken and chips surrounded by bell pepper and courgette slices, two veggies he did not eat. However, I guess he was feeling comfortable or brave, as he decided to give them a go. He tried both of them for the first time ever. He didn't initially think much of their taste (I think his taste buds are faulty) but it was a big step for him. He messaged his mom, proud of his accomplishment and since then, he accepts more and more veggies on his plate. Except tomatoes, I'm sure there's a story behind it! Not all his food stories have such happy ending though. We were travelling with a large group of people (that we didn't really know) and it was decided that that night we were going to cook a big meal for everyone to share at the hostel. We needed something easy to cook for a big number of people, so pasta was the obvious choice… Mike's worst nightmare. I remember him having his own separate meal which of course attracted curious eyes. I felt bad for him but I guess through experience he has learnt to adapt to these situations and realised it was better to keep to himself, and keep safe by eating what he was comfortable with.

Now Mike really enjoys cooking! He is slowly discovering the art of seasoning, spicing up his now almost daily eggs at breakfast, adding chilli flakes to our fajitas and is constantly widening his food palate. We try to make a point of buying something different at our weekly groceries. Or trying new appetizers when we go to the restaurant. I also noticed he is more open to trying new meals when travelling, I guess the adventurous feeling even affects his appetite.

Imagine my surprise when we had octopus and calamari in Greece! There is a clear gradual building up of confidence with time, which is important for me to encourage. Some aspects of his recovery he conquered brilliantly; food will be the next one. It must seem like I am making a big deal about this food stuff. But I think this really shows that Mike has come a long way, because if some small inconveniences are the biggest problems we face, considering everything else he has gone through, I think that's pretty good!

During these years of knowing Mike, there isn't much that has presented a real challenge to him – Crohn's wise. I often forget what is actually going on inside of him. Even if he doesn't show it, his body is constantly affected by the disease and is put under more pressure and receives more medication than most. I have never seen Mike go through a real flare up, never have seen him really suffer from his illness. I have never witnessed the full pain or seen the really ugly side of the disease, to me they are just stories, the same ones you read in this book. Yes, sad stories but ones we are now able to laugh at. So, even after knowing Mike for a long time and living with him, I don't fully understand how hard living with this uncurable illness can be.

So far, there has only been one situation where I have really felt the limitations of Mike's illness and have had to face the actual fragility of his condition in a way I had never experienced before. The COVID-19 outbreak in 2020. I know this probably brings some PTSD in all of us, but this truly exposed how quickly our normality could be taken away. For me COVID-19 would likely have been a simple viral infection, but it could have been much more severe for Mike. So in the very early stages of the pandemic, when I still went to work, I was extremely conscious of my surroundings and how letting my guard down for a moment could mean that I would be putting Mike's health at risk. The weeks prior to lockdown were very mentally draining for me, re-arranging my schedule to limit my exposure to other people and crowded spaces.

Eventually the UK government brought in lockdown and 'shielding'. For about three months, Mike and I weren't allowed to leave the flat under any circumstances. It was the first time that I felt so hopeless and so vulnerable. We were entirely dependent on others to do things for us, including bring us groceries. My mental health has never suffered so much, the thought of being prisoners in the tiny flat with no release date was terrifying. It was hard to accept that this was due to Mike's condition, which in my eyes, was not that limiting on our everyday life. But I knew that it was necessary to make sure that he was going to be ok. We managed to get through it, day by day, some most definitely harder than others, particularly for me as this type of isolation was totally new. Mike had already lived through similar isolation in his teens so he took it much better than me and he emotionally supported me throughout. He definitely was stronger and more focused during this time and his mental health suffered less than mine, which was a bit of a role reversal for us.

Depressive episodes are rare for Mike but not that rare. During the episodes he writes about, it is hard because I can never fully understand what triggers them or what is the best way to help, leaving me feeling powerless. I've learnt to not push too much, give him hugs when he needs them and try to get out of the house for some fresh air. There is certainly some psychological strain from his past years, as rarely can someone go through such series of events without repercussions on their mental health. But he has certainly managed this very well to this point without any medical help. As Mike explained, thankfully these are much less of an issue now, another battle he is winning – I continue to be so proud of him.

On the whole for us, Crohn's disease in no way impacts or defines our relationship. Any advice I could give can apply to any aspect of a relationship: be there for your partner, offer support and compassion when things get tougher, with open communication at the core. As mentioned, I fortunately haven't witnessed a fully blown Crohn's relapse thanks to the ileostomy bag, but if it ever does get worse, we both have the comfort of knowing that we can count on each other. I will never fully appreciate everything that Mike has been through, but the inevitable shaping of his character and the perspective of life it has given him has led to some amazing times together, always seeking new experiences and adventures.

www.ingramcontent.com/pod-product-compliance
Lightning Source LLC
Chambersburg PA
CBHW031156020426
42333CB00013B/700